Contents

House of Commons
Health Committee

Obesity

Third Report of Session 2003–04

Volume I

Report, together with formal minutes

*Ordered by The House of Commons
to be printed 10 May 2004*

HC 23-I
Published on 27 May 2004
by authority of the House of Commons
London: The Stationery Office Limited
£17.50

The Health Committee

The Health Committee is appointed by the House of Commons to examine the expenditure, administration, and policy of the Department of Health and its associated bodies.

Current membership

Mr David Hinchliffe MP (*Labour, Wakefield*) (Chairman)
Mr David Amess MP (*Conservative, Southend West*)
John Austin MP (*Labour, Erith and Thamesmead*)
Mr Keith Bradley MP (*Labour, Manchester Withington*)
Simon Burns MP (*Conservative, Chelmsford West*)
Mr Paul Burstow MP (*Liberal Democrat, Sutton and Cheam*)
Jim Dowd MP (*Labour, Lewisham West*)
Mr Jon Owen Jones MP (*Labour, Cardiff Central*)
Siobhain McDonagh MP (*Labour, Mitcham and Morden*)
Dr Doug Naysmith MP (*Labour, Bristol North West*)
Dr Richard Taylor MP (*Independent, Wyre Forest*)

The following Members were also members of the Committee in the course of this inquiry.
Mr Andy Burnham MP (*Labour, Leigh*)
Julia Drown MP (*Labour, South Swindon*)
Sandra Gidley MP (*Liberal Democrat, Romsey*)

Powers

The Committee is one of the departmental select committees, the powers of which are set out in House of Commons Standing Orders, principally in SO No 152. These are available on the Internet via www.parliament.uk.

Publications

The Reports and evidence of the Committee are published by The Stationery Office by Order of the House. All publications of the Committee (including press notices) are on the Internet at
www.parliament.uk/parliamentary_committees/health_committee.cfm.
A list of Reports of the Committee in the present Parliament is at the back of this volume.

Committee staff

The current staff of the Committee are Dr J S Benger (Clerk), Keith Neary (Second Clerk), Laura Hilder (Committee Specialist), Frank McShane (Committee Assistant) and Anne Browning (Secretary).

Contacts

All correspondence should be addressed to the Clerk of the Health Committee, House of Commons, 7 Millbank, London SW1P 3JA. The telephone number for general enquiries is 020 7219 6182. The Committee's email address is healthcom@parliament.uk .

Footnotes

In the footnotes of this Report, references to oral evidence are indicated by 'Q' followed by the question number. Written evidence is cited by reference to Volume II of this Report, in the form 'Ev' followed by the page number, and by reference to Appendix numbers for written evidence contained in Volume III.

Summary

Introduction

Around two-thirds of the population of England are overweight or obese. Obesity has grown by almost 400% in the last 25 years and on present trends will soon surpass smoking as the greatest cause of premature loss of life. It will entail levels of sickness that will put enormous strains on the health service. On some predictions, today's generation of children will be the first for over a century for whom life-expectancy falls.

Obesity is associated with many health problems including coronary heart disease, diabetes, kidney failure, osteoarthritis, back pain and psychological damage. The strong association between obesity and cancer has only recently come to light.

We estimate the economic costs of obesity conservatively at £3.3–3.7 billion per year and of obesity plus overweight at £6.6–7.4 billion.

Causes

Determining the causes of obesity is central to tackling it. The exact extent of the relative responsibility of diet and activity remains unclear and it is crucial that both sides of the 'energy equation' are addressed.

At its simplest level, obesity is caused when people overeat in relation to their energy needs. At the same time as energy expenditure has dropped considerably, environmental factors have combined to make it increasingly easy for people to consume more calories than they need. Energy-dense foods, which are highly calorific without being correspondingly filling, are becoming increasingly available. And while our evidence suggested that people are, generally speaking, aware of what constitutes a healthy diet, there are multiple barriers to their putting this into practice. In the absence of practical cookery lessons, children and young people are growing up without the skills to prepare healthy meals, compounding reliance on convenience foods, which are often high in energy density; healthy-eating messages are drowned out by the large proportion of advertising given over to highly energy-dense foods; other types of food promotion, as well as pricing also make buying unhealthy food more attractive and economical than healthy alternatives; and food labelling, a key tool to help consumers choose healthy foods, is frequently either confusing or absent.

Turning to the role of physical inactivity, only just over a third of men and around a quarter of women achieve the Department of Health's target of 30 minutes of physical activity 5 times a week. Levels of walking and cycling have fallen drastically in recent decades, while the number of cars has doubled in 30 years. Children are also increasingly sedentary both in and out of school. A fifth of boys and girls undertake less than 30 minutes activity a day. Television viewing has doubled since the 1960s, while physical activity is being squeezed out of daily life by the relentless march of automation.

Solutions

Solutions to the problem of obesity need to be multifaceted, recognising the true complexity of the issue, must address environmental as well as individual factors, and should be designed to bring about long-term, sustainable change, rather than promising overnight results. Obesity is also an issue which demands truly joined-up policy-making, and to ensure this we have recommended the appointment of a specific public health Cabinet committee, chaired by the Secretary of State for Health, to oversee the development of Public Service Agreement targets relating to obesity across all relevant government departments.

It is vital to ensure that the public are fully aware of the dangers of obesity and the importance of healthy eating, and that they also have the practical skills and information they need to implement these messages in their daily lives. To this end we have recommended a sustained public education campaign, improved practical food education for children and young people and, crucially, legislation to promote a simple food classification and labelling system which makes choosing healthy foods easy.

The promotional efforts of the food industry are frequently directed towards children. While we recognise that it is entirely appropriate for parents to retain control over their children's diet, we were shocked to find evidence that in its campaign for Walkers Wotsits, Abbot Mead Vickers advertising agency deliberately aimed to undermine parental control by exploiting 'pester power', despite this practice contravening the Advertising Standards Authority code of practice. We have recommended tighter controls on the advertising and promotion of foods to children, though we favour a voluntary approach in the first instance. We have also recommended that children's nutrition in school be improved, both through a move away from the promotion of high-energy density foods within schools, and through the introduction of better standards for school meals.

The Government has recently undertaken work with industry to reduce salt levels in foods, and we have recommended that work should be undertaken to reduce overall energy-density levels. We have also recommended that industry should undertake healthy pricing schemes, to make healthy foods a realistic choice for consumers who are buying food on a budget. Underpinning this, we believe that agricultural policies should also be reformed to take account of the public health agenda

Solutions to the problems of physical activity will demand a cohesive approach across many Government departments. We commend the funding and commitment now being devoted to organised recreation both in schools and in wider society though we note that fewer than half of school children are meeting the target of 2 hours of physical activity per week. This target itself we regard as inadequate and recommend instead a target of 3 hours physical activity a week for children. In order to involve those children traditionally 'turned off' sport we recommend that imaginative ways are found to broaden the physical activity agenda to include areas such as dance or aerobics. We also recommend that schools have in place effective strategies to counter bullying and elitism. Given the proven link between physical and academic achievement we recommend that Ofsted incorporates physical activity criteria in its school inspections.

Probably more important than organised recreation is the role of physical activity incorporated into the fabric of everyday life. We describe as scandalous the failure over 10 years of the Department for Transport to produce its promised walking strategy, and recommend that this is now included in a broader anti-obesity strategy. We also call on the Department of Health to have a strategic input into transport policy. We note the superior conditions for cyclists in other European countries, and whilst not offering detailed prescriptions for boosting cycling and walking levels, commend the Danish town planning we witnessed, notably in respect of proper segregation of cyclists and other road users. A key recommendation we make is for a health impact assessment to be made on major planning proposals which takes due account of the physical activity aspects.

We note the absence of evidence from business to our inquiry and call on the Government to generate awareness of obesity in the business community and on the Treasury to consider fiscal incentives to make the workplace more active.

While environmental solutions are clearly key to tackling obesity at a population level, we also feel that the NHS has an important role to play, both in the prevention and treatment of obesity, but our evidence suggests that this has not been as high a priority for PCTs as it should have been. We have heard of GPs being asked to limit the prescription of NICE-approved obesity drugs, of specialist obesity services with closed waiting lists, and of pioneering local projects threatened with closure due to lack of funding. To address this, we have recommended the establishment of a strategic framework for preventing and treating obesity within the NHS, drawing on existing National Service Frameworks. This should be underpinned by stringent public health targets, and must include the expansion of services to treat obese patients within both primary and secondary care. A full range of treatment options should be open to obese patients, including behavioural or lifestyles approaches, counselling, drug therapy, and, as a last resort, surgery. In particular, children must have access to appropriate services, and should be screened for overweight and obesity annually within a school setting.

Conclusion

In conclusion we note that it is difficult to establish the impact of any individual measure to combat so complex and challenging an issue as obesity; this is not, in our view, an excuse to delay and measures must be taken to tackle the nation's diet and its levels of activity. We acknowledge the responsibility of the individual in respect of his or her own health but believe that the Government must resist inaction caused by political anxiety over accusations of "nanny statism". Government will, after all, have to pay for some of the huge costs that will accrue if the epidemic of obesity goes unchecked. While we have tried wherever possible to take the food industry at its word, and seen it as 'part of the solution', we recommend that the Government reviews the situation in three years and then decides if more direct regulation is required.

1 Introduction

1. With quite astonishing rapidity, an epidemic of obesity has swept over England. To describe what has happened as an epidemic may seem far-fetched. That word is normally applied to a contagious disease that is rapidly spreading. But the proportion of the population that is obese has grown by almost 400% in the last 25 years. Around two-thirds of the population are now overweight or obese. On present trends, obesity will soon surpass smoking as the greatest cause of premature loss of life. It will bring levels of sickness that will put enormous strains on the health service, perhaps even making a publicly funded health service unsustainable.

2. Dr Sheila McKenzie, a consultant at the Royal London Hospital which recently opened an obesity service for children, offered a powerful insight into the crisis posed to the nation's health. Despite only being in existence for three years, her service had an eleven-month waiting list. Over the last two years, she had witnessed a child of three dying from heart failure where extreme obesity was a contributory factor. Four of the children in the care of her unit were being managed at home with non-invasive ventilatory assistance for sleep apnoea: as she put it, "in other words, they are choking on their own fat."[1]

3. A generation is growing up in an obesogenic environment in which the forces behind sedentary behaviour are growing, not declining. Most overweight or obese children become overweight or obese adults; overweight and obese adults are more likely to bring up overweight or obese children. There is little encouraging evidence to suggest that overweight people generally lose weight; there is ample clear evidence that being overweight greatly increases the risks of a huge range of diseases, and that the more overweight people are, the greater the risks. Yet paradoxically, the phenomenal increase in weight comes at a time when there is an apparent obsession with personal appearance. There are more gyms than ever, more options presented as 'healthy eating', and the Atkins diet dominates the best seller charts.

4. Little has been done to reverse trends in obesity. According to Professor Sir George Alberti, President of the International Diabetes Federation, this is partly because the phenomenon has "insidiously crept in" and partly because it raises politically sensitive issues.[2] Dr Geof Rayner, then Chair of the UK Public Health Association, suggested that another issue was the sheer difficulty in knowing how to combat obesity: "when you have big explanations which you cannot pinpoint exactly then it is very difficult to see what you can do about it."[3] For Professor Julian Peto, Head of Epidemiology at the Institute of Cancer Research, another reason for the neglect was the fact that some of the health risks of obesity had not been known for long. In particular, the extent of the link with cancer had only recently emerged following a major US cohort study.[4] Professor Hubert Lacey, for the Royal College of Psychiatrists, argued that part of the problem was stigma and prejudice

---

1   Appendix 33

2   Q170

3   Q172

4   Q172

against the obese, both within society at large and within the medical profession: "as a group clinically they are not liked … [they are seen as having] brought it on themselves."[5]

5. So rapid has been the rise in obesity that there is a danger it will overtake the population to the extent that what used to be considered 'overweight' starts to become 'normal'. Moreover, as Professor Peto pointed out, "the NHS cannot provide detailed clinical services or intensive clinical services" for the 20% of the population who are obese, and amongst whom two-thirds of the excessive mortality occurs.[6]

6. Society is rapidly changing to absorb the trend in weight. One American airline has started charging obese passengers for two seats.[7] A woman was recently awarded £13,000 compensation from Virgin Atlantic, after developing a large bruise, and muscle and nerve damage which made her bedridden for a month, caused by being wedged next to an obese female passenger for an 11 hour flight.[8] A recent study in Leeds suggested that schoolchildren now require trousers two sizes larger than did their counterparts only 20 years ago.[9] Another report has concluded that 23.6% of British children under four are overweight, compared with 14.7% ten years earlier. A major re-insurance firm has just completed a study concluding that the obese will soon have to pay larger premiums.[10] In America, super-size coffins are now available, and burial plot sizes are increasing.[11]

7. It is often said that Britain lags behind America by a few years in cultural patterns. Trends in obesity in Britain do indeed follow, albeit with a delay of a few years, those in America. And such are the trends in obesity in that country that it is now predicted that one in three American children will eventually become diabetic, which in itself will pose an almost unimaginable disease and cost burden on that country.[12]

8. The Chief Medical Officer has referred to obesity as "a health time bomb" that needs defusing.[13] He noted the World Health Organization (WHO) prediction that the world will "see a one-third increase in the loss of healthy life as a result of overweight and obesity over the next 20 years, with the number of global deaths rising from three million to five million each year."

9. The WHO itself describes an escalating global epidemic of overweight and obesity— "globesity"—that is taking over many parts of the world. In their view, "If immediate action is not taken, millions will suffer from an array of serious health disorders."[14]

---

5   Q172, 185

6   Q195

7   *The Times*, 24 Feb 2004

8   *Sunday Times*, 20 October 2002

9   M.C.J. Rudolf et al, "Rising obesity and expanding waistlines in schoolchildren: a cohort study", *Archives of Disease in Childhood*, 89 (2004), pp 235-37

10   *The Guardian*, 7 April 2004

11   *Scotland on Sunday*, 5 October 2003

12   Centers for Disease Control Report presented to 63rd Annual Society, American Diabetes Association

13   Annual Report of the Chief Medical Officer 2002

14   See www.who.int/nut/obs.htm.

10. Should the gloomier scenarios relating to obesity turn out to be true, the sight of amputees will become much more familiar in the streets of Britain. There will be many more blind people. There will be huge demand for kidney dialysis. The positive trends of recent decades in combating heart disease, partly the consequence of the decline in smoking, will be reversed. Indeed, "this will be the first generation where children die before their parents as a consequence of childhood obesity."[15]

Scope and nature of our inquiry

11. We announced our intention of holding an inquiry into obesity on 28 March 2003 with the following terms of reference:

The inquiry will cover:
The health implications of obesity
What are the health outcomes of obesity in society? What are the economic and social costs? What efforts is the Government making to evaluate these?
Trends in obesity
What are the trends in obesity (including trends among particular groups, by social class, age, gender, ethnicity and lifestyle)? What is the relationship between obesity and other health inequalities? What are the international comparisons (EU, OECD, USA)?
What are the causes of the rise in obesity in recent decades?
What has been the role of changes in diet? To what extent have changes in lifestyle, particularly moves to a more sedentary lifestyle, been influential? How much is lack of physical activity contributing to the problem?
What can be done about it?
What is the range of 'levers' and drivers (food industry, marketing, education, family life, genetics, drugs, surgery)? Within that range, what role can the food industry, marketing and advertising, transport and schooling play? What are the responsibilities of the food industry in respect of marketing? How influential is the media? How can the amount of physical activity being undertaken be increased? To what extent can and should Government, at central and local level, influence lifestyle choices? How coherent is national and local strategy? What is international best practice?
Are the institutional structures in place to deliver an improvement?
What is the role of the Department of Health (DoH) and of the NHS, including that of primary care, hospitals and specialist clinics? How effective are the structures for health promotion? Can health promotion compete with huge food sector advertising budgets? To what extent can the food industry be part of a solution? To what extent is the Food Standards Agency influential? How well is the DoH liaising with, and what is the role of, other central and local government departments and bodies? What is the role of schools, including sport in schools? Who should 'own' and drive delivery? Have we the appropriate institutional structures, budgets and priorities?
Recommendations for national and local strategy
How can the Government's strategy be improved? What are the policy options? Can they be better integrated? What are the priorities for action?

---

15   Appendix 4 (Dr Mary Rudolf); this point was recently echoed by the Chair of the Food Standards Agency. See *The Observer,* 9 November 2003.

12. Since 12 June 2003 we have taken oral evidence on no fewer than 14 occasions making this the most comprehensive inquiry the Health Committee has ever undertaken. We have heard from: Ministers and officials in the Departments of Health (hereafter 'the Department'), Culture, Media and Sport (DCMS), and Education and Skills (DfES); officials from the Food Standards Agency (FSA), the Office of the Deputy Prime Minister (ODPM), the Department for Environment, Food and Rural Affairs (DEFRA) and the Department for Transport; representatives of fast food, carbonated drinks, breakfast cereals and confectionery companies and the advertising agencies representing them; major supermarkets; epidemiologists; experts on obesity, the food industry and physical activity; health professionals; Mr Barry Gardiner MP (who has pioneered a scheme extending the school day to incorporate greater physical activity); and Professor Marion Nestle, Chair of the Department of Nutrition, Food Studies and Public Health, New York University.

13. We received around 150 memoranda from health professionals, representatives of the food industry, academics, advertisers, commercial slimming organizations, those working in sport, recreation and physical activity, and members of the public.

14. We are extremely grateful to all those who submitted written and oral evidence to our inquiry. We are also very grateful to our five specialist advisers: Dr Laurel Edmunds, Senior Researcher for the Avon Longitudinal Study of Parents and Children, University of Bristol; Professor Ken Fox, Department of Exercise and Health Sciences, University of Bristol; Professor Gerard Hastings, Director, Centre for Social Marketing and Centre for Tobacco Control Research, University of Strathclyde; Professor Phil James, Director of the Rowett Research Institute, Aberdeen and Chair of the International Obesity Taskforce; and Tim Lang, Professor of Food Policy, City University. This has been a contentious inquiry, with powerful interest groups carefully watching our work. We are grateful for the objective and expert support we have received from our advisers. We are also very grateful to the Clerk's Department Scrutiny Unit, who provided us with an extremely helpful analysis of the economic costs of obesity, which is annexed to this report. We should also like to thank Liz Powell-Bullock and Adriana Rodriguez for supplementary research for this report.

15. The USA is experiencing particularly disastrous trends in obesity and we wanted to see at first hand what the scale of the problem was and what measures were being taken to address it. Accordingly, in October 2003 we visited the USA. In New York, we met Dr Xavier Pi-Sunyer, a world expert in diabetes at the Obesity Research Center; we visited the Strang Cancer Prevention Center; we met doctors at the New York Presbyterian Hospital, including a representative from the Comprehensive Weight Control Center; we received a presentation from Dr Christine Ren and Dr George Fielding, bariatric surgeons;[16] we met representatives of the New York City Parks Department; finally, we held discussions with Fleishman-Hillard Marketing and Professor Marion Nestle.

16. In Atlanta, Georgia we held discussions with a range of experts from the Centers for Disease Control; we met senior representatives of Coca-Cola; and then met Dr David Satcher, the former Surgeon General of the United States and Director of the Morehouse School of Medicine.

---

16   Bariatric surgery is surgery on the stomach and/or intestines to help patients with extreme obesity lose weight.

17. Finally we visited Denver, Colorado which leads the national strategy to counter obesity through physical activity, and is the leanest state in America. Here we met representatives of the Colorado Physical Activity and Nutrition Program, the Department of Education, the Healthy Foods/Five-a-day project and the Department of Transportation. We also met Dr James Hill, Director of the America on the Move project, and representatives of Colorado on the Move.

18. Since the EU has a locus in public health in member nations we visited Brussels in December 2003. Here we met David Byrne, EU Commissioner for Health and Consumer Protection, and officials, Mr Andrew Hayes from the International Union against Cancer and the Association of European Cancer Leagues, representatives of the Confederation of the Food and Drink Industries of the EU, and representatives of the European Heart Network.

19. We also visited Finland and Denmark in connection with this and other inquiries. Although Finland experienced substantial growth in obesity in the 1980s and 1990s it has been successful in greatly reducing death through coronary heart disease and has, as a nation, altered its diet and boosted its exercise levels. Although Finland has not managed to reverse the overall growth of obesity, it has managed to reduce the steepness of the curve in trends in obesity in men, and flatten it entirely in women. Finland now has obesity rates lower than England for both males and females. We wanted to see at first hand how it had succeeded in doing that. Denmark has recently agreed a national obesity strategy which could offer many parallels to England.

20. In Finland, we met the Minister for Public Health and officials in the Ministry of Social Affairs and Health, staff and pupils in Pikku Huopalathi school, the National Public Health Institute, Professor Aila Risannen and staff at Helsinki University Central Hospital, and members of the Parliamentary Social Affairs and Health Committee.

21. In Denmark we met officials from the Ministry for the National Board of Health, including the Chief Medical Officer; we also visited the town of Odense which has a particularly advanced transport system, integrating cycle and pedestrian travel.

22. Within England, we undertook a visit to Leeds to witness a specialist obesity clinic, and went to a range of primary and secondary schools to look at physical activity and sport in schools and school meals. We also held informal discussions there with a wide range of health and education professionals. We also visited Bradford Bulls Rugby League Football Club, which has an excellent community outreach scheme, involving children in health education and physical activity.

23. We are extremely grateful to all those, including the Foreign and Commonwealth Office staff, who facilitated these visits which offered crucial evidence to our inquiry, on which we have drawn considerably in formulating this report.

Defining obesity

24. According to the Faculty of Public Health, obesity is "an excess of body fat frequently resulting in a significant impairment of health and longevity."[17] Body fatness is most

commonly assessed by body mass index (BMI) which is calculated by dividing an individual's weight measured in kilogrammes by their height in metres squared. We annex, at Annex 2, a chart which will allow readers of this report to calculate their own BMI. Overweight is generally defined as a BMI greater than 25; individuals with a BMI greater than 30 are classified as obese:

Table 1: Classification of Body Mass Index and Risk of Co-morbidities

Classification	BMI (kg/m^2)	Risk of co-morbidities
Underweight	<18.5	Low (but risk of other clinical problems increased)
Normal range	18.5–24.9	Average
Overweight	25.0–29.9	Mildly increased
Obese	**>30.0**	
Class I	30.0–34.9	Moderate
Class II	35.0–39.9	Severe
Class III severe (or 'morbid obesity' or 'super obesity')	>40.0	Very severe

Source: International Obesity Task Force

25. It is important to recognise that obesity is both a medical condition and a lifestyle disorder and both factors have to be seen within a context of individual, family and societal functioning.

26. There is no generally agreed definition of childhood obesity but two widely favoured indicators are based respectively on percentiles of UK reference curves (85th centile for overweight, 95th centile for obesity) and on reference points derived from an international (six country) survey.[18]

27. The correlations between BMI and the risk of co-morbidities in the table above offer a good summary of the situation but also oversimplify it. For example, individuals of South Asian descent have an increased risk of obesity-related disorders, triggered at lower BMI ratios than those above, but this is not taken into account in the current guidelines for obesity management. A BMI of 27.5 or more in an Asian person has been estimated to be associated with comparable morbidities to those in a Caucasian person with a BMI of 30.[19]

28. Central obesity, that is to say a high waist:hip ratio, is another measurement used to define obesity. Central obesity is sometimes defined as a waist:hip ratio greater than 0.95 in

---

18 In 1990 a nationally representative sample of children had their heights and weights measured. The resulting BMIs were used to generate the UK standard reference charts. The range of BMIs for each sex and age was divided into 100 parts or centiles. For example the 50th centile represents the average BMI, the 3rd centile provides the level at which the thinnest 3% of the population would be identified and similarly, the 97th centile identified the most overweight 3% of the population. Therefore the 85th centile identified the top 15% overweight in the population and 95th the top 5% as obese.

19 World Health Organization expert consultation cited in Royal College of Physicians, *Storing up problems: the medical cure for a slimmer nation* (2004), p3.

men and 0.85 in women. A simpler indicator used in a WHO report is that increased risk is present when the waist circumference exceeds 37 inches for men or 32 inches for women.[20]

How prevalent is obesity?

29. Professor Terence Wilkin, of Peninsula University Plymouth, pointed out that over the past 30 years the median body mass of the population has risen as fast as the mean, "suggesting that society is getting fatter, not just those who are already fat."[21]

30. The Health of the Nation targets in 1992 were for fewer than 6% of men and 8% of women to be obese by 2005.[22] The latest figures make disturbing reading, and the trend data show how obesity has more than trebled in the last two decades. These figures are from the Department's own memorandum, updated to take account of data taken from the Health Survey for 2002:

Table 2: Prevalence of obesity in England 1980–2002

Men

Body Mass Index	1980	1993	2000	2002
	%	%	%	%
Healthy weight: 20–25		37.8	29.9	29.6
Overweight: 25–30		44.4	44.5	43.4
Obese: Over 30	6	13.2	21.0	22.1
Morbidly obese: Over 40		0.2	0.6	0.8

Women

Body Mass Index	1980	1993	2000	2002
	%	%	%	%
Healthy weight: 20–25		44.3	39.0	37.4
Overweight: 25–30		32.2	33.8	33.7
Obese: Over 30	8	16.4	21.4	22.8
Morbidly obese: Over 40		1.4	2.3	2.6

Source: Department of Health (Ev 3) and Health Survey for England 2002

31. Amongst children, one study found that obesity and overweight showed little change between 1974 and 1984, but between 1984 and 1994 overweight increased from 5.4% to 9% in English boys and from 9.3% to 13.5% in girls; the prevalence of obesity reached 1.7% in

---

20   Cited in National Audit Office (NAO), *Tackling Obesity in England* (2001), p11.

21   Appendix 37

22   Cited in Appendix 18 (Royal College of General Practitioners).

boys and 2.6% in girls.[23] The 2002 Health Survey for England noted a substantial deterioration in the decade subsequent to this study:

> About one in 20 boys (5.5%) and about one in 15 girls (7.2%) aged 2–15 were obese in 2002, according to the International classification. Overall, over one in five boys (21.8%) and over one in four girls (27.5%) were either overweight or obese. In comparison with the International classification, obesity estimates derived by the National BMI percentiles classification were much higher (16.0% for boys and 15.9% for girls). The difference between the two estimates is small for girls when the combined overweight including obesity category is considered (30.7% vs 27.5%), but remains more marked for boys (30.3% vs 21.8%). About one in ten young men (9.2%) and women (11.5%) were obese, while about one in three young men (32.2%) and young women (32.8%) were overweight or obese.[24]

32. Projecting these figures forwards by 15 years simply by assuming a steady growth suggests that around one-third of adults will be obese by 2020. However, "if the rapid acceleration in childhood obesity in the last decade is taken into account, the predicted prevalence in children for 2020 will be in excess of 50%."[25]

33. The following table lists the prevalence of obesity (defined as BMI above 30) in various European countries:

23   Susan Chinn and Roberto Rona, "Prevalence and trends in overweight and obesity in three cross sectional studies of British children," 1974–94, *British Medical Journal* 322 (2001), pp 24-26

24   Department of Health, Health Survey for England 2002

25   RCP, *Storing up problems*, p4

Figure 1: Obesity levels in Europe

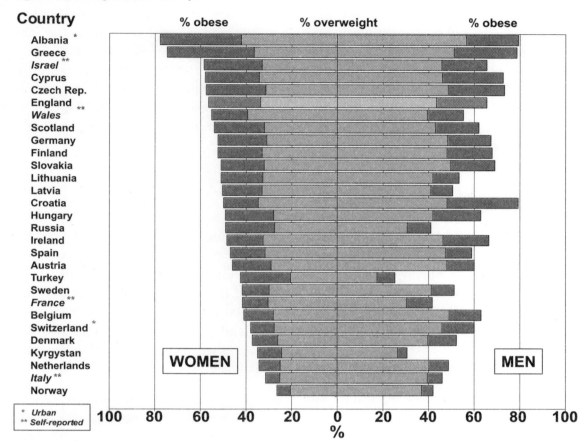

Source: International Obesity Task Force

34. Not only does England have some of the worst figures in Europe but it also demonstrates some of the worst trends in the acceleration of obesity: in the majority of European countries the prevalence of obesity has increased between 10–40% in the last ten years, but in England it has more than doubled.

35. In 1995, according to the WHO, there were an estimated 200 million obese adults worldwide and another 18 million children aged under five classified as overweight.[26] However, by 2000, the number of obese adults had increased to over 300 million.

36. Contrary to conventional wisdom, the obesity epidemic is not restricted to industrialised societies. Some 115 million people suffer from obesity-related problems in the non-industrialised world. For example:

- Over three-quarters of men living in cities in Samoa are obese;

- There are as many overweight as underweight adults in Ghana;

- 44% of women in the Cape Peninsula of South Africa are obese.[27]

---

26   www.who/int/nut

27   International Obesity Taskforce—see www.iotf.org .

37. There is enormous variation in obesity rates even within countries with the highest GDPs. The USA is near the top of any table of obesity rates but Japan is nearer the bottom. Despite the entry of US-style eating chains in Japan, its food culture has proved sufficiently robust so far to resist some of the global trends in obesity. This cultural dimension is important: obesity should not be seen as an inevitable result of economic advance. However, it is true to say that, as countries develop, there is a marked shift in the proportion of the population who are overweight as opposed to underweight. Ironically, in many countries the problem of malnutrition is being superseded or complemented by the problem of obesity.

Obesity and health inequalities

38. In common with most public health problems the impact of obesity mirrors many other health inequalities. Men and women working in unskilled manual occupations are over four times as likely as those in professional employment to be classified as morbidly obese.[28] The Health Survey for England has shown that in 2001 amongst professional groups 14% of men and women were obese, compared to 28% of women and 19% of men in unskilled manual occupations.[29] Children who are Asian are four times more likely to be obese than those who are white.[30] Pakistani, Indian and Bangladeshi men have relatively low levels of obesity measured by BMI, but 41% of Indian men are classed as centrally obese compared to 28% of men in the general population.[31]

39. Amongst women, there are also important differences between ethnic groups: in 1999 obesity was 50% higher than the national average amongst Black Caribbean women and 25% higher amongst Pakistani women.

What are the potential health risks of obesity and what are the costs of these?

40. There is a nine-year reduction in life expectancy amongst obese patients, the risk being markedly amplified if they also smoke. Generalised obesity (fat distributed around the whole body) results in alterations in the blood circulation and heart function, while central/abdominal obesity (fatness mainly around the chest and abdomen) further restricts chest movements and alters breathing function. Fat around the abdomen is also a major contributor to the development of diabetes, hypertension, and alterations in blood lipid (fat and cholesterol) concentrations.[32]

41. Overweight and obesity are associated with a wide range of conditions as the table below shows:

---

28   Appendix 5 (British Medical Foundation)

29   Chief Medical Officer's Report, 2002

30   Appendix 29 (Medical Research Council)

31   Ev 115

32   *Storing up problems*, p 7

Table 3: Relative risks of health problems associated with obesity[33]

Greatly increased (relative risk much greater than 3)	Moderately increased (relative risk 2–3)	Slightly increased (relative risk 1–2)
Type 2 diabetes	Coronary Heart Disease	Cancer (breast cancer in postmenopausal women, endometrial cancer, colon cancer)
Gallbladder disease	Hypertension	Reproductive hormone abnormalities
Dyslipidaemia	Osteoarthritis (Knees)	Polycystic ovary syndrome
Insulin resistance	Hyperuricaemia and gout	Impaired fertility
Breathlessness		Low back pain
Sleep apnoea		Anaesthetic risk
		Fetal defects associated with maternal obesity

Source: WHO (1998)

42. According to the 2002 WHO World Health Report: "Overweight and obesity lead to adverse metabolic effects on blood pressure, cholesterol, triglycerides[34] and insulin resistance. Risks of coronary heart disease, ischaemic stroke and type 2 diabetes mellitus increase steadily with increasing BMI." Raised BMI also "increases the risk of cancer of the breast, colon, prostate, endometrium, kidney and gallbladder."[35]

43. In non-smokers, the relative risk of death has been estimated to rise in relation to increased body weight by the following factors:

Table 4: Classification of Body Mass Index and Relative Risk of Death

BMI	Relative risk of death
25–26.9	1.3
27–28.9	1.6
29–31	2.1

Source: RCGP (Appendix 18)

44. Overweight and obesity are regarded as amongst the main modifiable risks associated with **coronary heart disease (CHD) and cardio-vascular disease generally**. The British Heart Foundation estimates that around 5% of CHD deaths in men and 6% in women are due to obesity as such[36] and a higher proportion if the large number of overweight adults is also considered.

45. Perhaps the most dramatic impact has come in the area of **diabetes**. Already there are over two million diabetics living in the UK (only around half of whom will have had the disease diagnosed); that figure is projected to rise to three million by 2010.[37] Worldwide, the number of diabetics is projected to rise from 200 to 300 million over the period 2000 to 2020.[38] The prevalence of diabetes has increased by 65% in men and 25% in women since

---

33　All relative risk estimates are approximate. The relative risk indicates the risk measured against that of a non-obese person. For example, an obese person is two to three times more likely to suffer from hypertension than is a non-obese person.

34　Triglycerides are blood fats.

35　WHO, World Health Report 2002, p 60

36　Appendix 5

37　Appendix 23 (Diabetes UK)

38　Appendix 3; Q216 (Professor Alberti)

1991.[39] It represents a massive and growing threat to public health, given that typically the gap between onset and diagnosis of the disease is 9–12 years. Already, some 20% of the South Asian population is diabetic and 25% are glucose-intolerant, a precursor condition for diabetes. On some projections, by 2025 diabetes could account for a quarter of the health budget.[40]

46. Obesity triggers a state of insulin resistance. Professor Terence Wilkin, from Peninsula University, Plymouth, and Director of the Early Bird Study which seeks to establish the factors in childhood that lead to insulin resistance and diabetes, suggested that hyperinsulinaemia drives a host of metabolic disturbances besides diabetes:

> [these are known as:] the metabolic syndrome, and include hypertension, hypercholesterolaemia, hypertriglyceridaemia, hypercoagulation, hyperviscosity and hyperuricaemia. Each in itself is a risk factor for coronary artery disease, but together they are catastrophic—the so-called syndrome X [or metabolic syndrome].[41]

47. Professor Wilkin concluded that, rather than being a "complication" of diabetes, premature cardiovascular disease is an "inevitable association" of the condition.

48. Whereas type 2 diabetes was hitherto normally associated with diabetes developing in adults over the age of 35—it was often termed "late onset" or "adult onset" diabetes—it is increasingly being diagnosed in children.[42] One estimate suggests that up to 45% of cases of diabetes diagnosed in children in the USA are now type 2.[43] As Professor A H Barnett, Clinical Director for Diabetes and Endocrine Services at the University of Birmingham, noted: "figures from the USA … indicate a very serious long-term outlook for these children, with significant numbers dying from heart attack or being on kidney dialysis and/or blind before the age of 40 years."[44] Dr Tim Barrett, a paediatrician at Birmingham Children's Hospital, told us that it was only since about the year 2000 that the medical profession had started seeing children with type 2 diabetes in England, but that this disease now accounted for about 6% of the children attending his clinic with diabetes. The youngest patient he had seen, who had developed some symptoms, was a super-obese eight year old girl.[45]

49. The progress of diabetes is so closely entwined with that of obesity that in America it has produced the coinage "diabesity".[46] Diabetes leads to cardio-vascular problems, and can also entail blindness following damage to the small blood vessels of the eye, kidney failure, stroke, osteoarthritis, and damage to the nervous system which can lead to leg ulcers and limb amputation. A long-term study of 51 Canadian patients aged 18–33 years diagnosed with type 2 diabetes before the age of 17 years found that:

---

39 Ev 115 (National Heart Forum)

40 Appendix 3 (Professor A Barnett)

41 Appendix 37

42 Type 1 diabetes used to be known as "juvenile diabetes". It is an auto-immune disease, now representing less than 10% of diabetes world-wide.

43 A Pagota Campagna, "Emergence of type 2 diabetes mellitus in children: epidemiological evidence", *Journal Paediatric Endocrinology and Metabolism* 13 (2000), supplement 6, pp 1395-1402

44 Appendix 3

45 Q195

46 *The Guardian*, 10 May 2003, "Food: The way we eat now", p17

Seven had died; three others were on dialysis; one became blind at the age of 26; and one had had a toe amputation. Of 56 pregnancies in this cohort, only 35 had resulted in live births (62.5%).[47]

50. Children contracting type 2 diabetes will also have a life-time to develop the severe sequelae of the disease and their diabetes is much more difficult to control than those children developing the classic form of type 1 diabetes with insulin deficiency.

51. It is crucial to realise that for diabetes—and indeed many of the conditions listed here—it is not necessary to be *obese* to increase the risk of morbidity. Risks rapidly accelerate as people become *overweight*. As Professor Andrew Prentice, Head of the Medical Research Council's International Nutrition Group at the London School of Hygiene and Tropical Medicine, noted, "If you look at the risks for diabetes … [in] people with a BMI that does not classify them as clinically obese (a BMI of around 28 in women) the increased risk of diabetes is 18-fold."[48] But risks continue to accelerate as BMI grows. According to Professor Sir George Alberti, President of the International Diabetes Federation, a study of nurses in the USA has revealed that those with a BMI of 35 had "a 92-fold increase in risk of diabetes" compared with those with a BMI of 22.[49]

52. Diabetes is also associated with health inequalities: diabetes is three to five times more common in people of African and Caribbean origin living in the UK.[50]

53. Professor A H Barnett estimated that diabetes "now costs the Exchequer around 9% of the total healthcare budget of the UK, with projections that by 2025 that this could reach 25% of the total healthcare budget."[51]

54. **End-stage renal failure** is a complication of diabetes. According to the National Kidney Federation, renal failure is set to increase massively: yet already services in the UK are "overwhelmed" in terms of capacity and financial resources.[52]

55. Around 14% of **cancer** deaths in men and 20% in women are attributed to obesity.[53] Obesity is associated with breast, endometrial, oesophageal and colonic cancers.[54] According to Professor Julian Peto, for the Institute of Cancer Research, obesity is "far and away the most important avoidable cause" of cancer in non-smokers.[55] Cancer Research UK suggested that 1 in 7 cancer deaths in men and 1 in 5 in women in the USA, are attributable to overweight and obesity. This implies that 1 in 8 UK cancer deaths are thus caused. The clear association between obesity and cancer, in the view of the charity, is

---

47 H Dean and B Flett, "Natural History of type 2 diabetes diagnosed in childhood: long term follow-up in young adult years", *Diabetes* 2002:51 (suppl 2) A24-25, cited in RCP, *Storing up problems: the medical case for a slimmer nation*, 2004, p 8; Q195 (Dr Barrett)

48 Q362

49 Q174

50 Appendix 23 (Diabetes UK)

51 Appendix 3; see further C J Currie et al, "NHS acute sector expenditure for diabetes: the present, future and excess in-patient cost of care," *Diabetic Medicine*, 14 (1997), pp 686-92

52 Appendix 1

53 Appendix 11 (UK Association for the Study of Obesity)

54 Q174; Q178

55 Q210

"poorly acknowledged outside the scientific community".[56] A recent survey showed that only 3% of the population was aware of the link between overweight and cancer even though this factor is the main preventable risk factor after tobacco use, and will eventually become the main risk factor.[57] Professor Peto cited a Framingham study which suggested that in female non-smokers who are obese life expectancy is seven years shorter.[58]

56. The National Obesity Forum presented evidence to suggest that around 20 different cancers have been linked to obesity. They also noted that in the morbidly obese, death rates from cancer were 52% higher for men and 60% higher for women.[59]

57. **Osteoarthritis**, a joint disorder which typically affects the joints in knees, hips, and lower back, is exacerbated by overweight. Weight gain appears to increase the risk of osteoarthritis by placing extra pressure on these joints and wearing away the protective cartilage. **Back pain**, one of the commonest health problems caused or exacerbated by overweight and obesity, leads to more than 11 million lost working days each year in Britain.[60]

58. **Psychological damage** caused by overweight and obesity is a huge health burden. In childhood, the first problems caused are likely to be emotional and psychological.[61] Moreover, the psychological consequences of obesity can range from lowered self-esteem to clinical depression. Rates of anxiety and depression are three to four times higher among obese individuals.[62] Obese women are around 37% more likely to commit suicide than women of normal weight.[63]

59. The seminal 2001 National Audit Office (NAO) Report, *Tackling Obesity in England*, noted:

> Obese people … are more likely to suffer from a number of psychological problems, including binge-eating, low self-image and confidence, and a sense of isolation and humiliation arising from practical problems.[64]

60. Professor Hubert Lacey, for the Royal College of Psychiatrists, told us that depression tended to be caused by obesity, rather than obesity by depression:

> There is not a clear link between massive obesity and a pre-existing psychological problem; rather there is evidence of psychological sequelae from the massive obesity itself.[65]

---

56   Ev 57

57   NOP poll for Cancer Research UK. See BBC News UK, 5 April 2004.

58   Q212

59   Ev 318

60   BBC health website at www.bbc.co.uk

61   Appendix 20 (Royal College of Paediatrics and Child Health)

62   IOTF website at www.iotf.org

63   Appendix 6 (Roche)

64   *Tackling Obesity in England*, p 56

65   Q182

This professional analysis is the opposite of that held by the public and indeed by many doctors.

61. Excess weight is also likely to lead to prejudice in the workplace, lower self-esteem and reduced job opportunities. According to Professor Jane Wardle, of the Health Behaviour Unit at University College London, a recent study has demonstrated that teachers underestimate the IQ of overweight children.[66]

62. One recent study has concluded that "Mortality attributable to excess weight is a major public health problem in the EU. At least one in 13 annual deaths in the EU are likely to be related to excess weight." However, in that figure the UK has the highest individual percentage of all, with 8.7% of deaths being attributable to excess weight.[67]

What are the economic costs?

63. The NAO estimated that the direct cost of treating obesity and its consequences in 1998 was £480 million (1.5% of NHS expenditure) and that indirect costs (loss of earnings due to sickness and premature mortality) amounted to £2.1 billion, giving an overall total of £2.58 billion. A total projected figure of £3.6 billion was given for 2010. Although these figures have been widely quoted in much subsequent work on obesity, the authors consistently acknowledge the conservative nature of their estimates.[68]

64. We asked the House of Commons Clerk's Department Scrutiny Unit to revisit the NAO calculations and analyse them so as to produce a more up-to-date and comprehensive analysis of the costs of obesity. Their work is annexed to this report at Annex 1.

65. However, in summary the findings of the Scrutiny Unit were as follows:

- The calculations of the cost of obesity made in the NAO report *Tackling Obesity in England* are said to be conservative and underestimates by its authors.

- Estimates of the cost of obesity from other countries are nearly all well above those for England, as a proportion of healthcare spending, even though obesity levels were generally lower.

- The direct cost of treating obesity in England in 2002 is estimated at £46–49 million.

- The costs of treating the consequences of obesity are an estimated £945–1,075 million.

- The indirect costs of obesity in 2002 are estimated at £1–1.1 billion for premature mortality and £1.3–1.45 billion for sickness absence.

66. **The Clerk's Department Scrutiny Unit has recalculated the total estimated cost of obesity is therefore £3.3–3.7 billion. This is £0.7–1.1 billion (27–42%) more than the NAO estimate for 1998. The difference between the two figures occurs for a number of**

---

66 Q189

67 See J R Banegas et al, "A simple estimate of mortality attributable to excess weight in the European Union", *European Journal of Clinical Nutrition*, 57 (2003), pp 201-8.

68 *Tackling Obesity in England*, para 2.27; see also appendix 6 paras 17-18, 22, 25, 28 and 33-34.

reasons including higher NHS and drug costs, more accurate data that have been produced recently, the inclusion of more co-morbidities and the increased prevalence of obesity. This figure should still be regarded as an under-estimate. We note that these analyses are for the 20% of the adult population who are already obese. If in crude terms the costs of being overweight are on average only half of those of being obese then, with more than twice as many overweight as obese men and women, these costs would double. This would yield an overall cost estimate for overweight and obesity of £6.6–7.4 billion per year.

2 Causes

What has happened in our environment in terms of the history of human evolution is remarkable in the last two generations. We have never seen anything like this, where we have the coming together of the technological, electronic, television revolution and the highly available, high energy-dense and very cheap foods ... where physical activity comes in is that you rapidly get into a vicious cycle of inactivity, sloth and weight gain: as soon as you start to gain a load of weight, it is all the more difficult to go up those stairs; as soon as you start to become a little less fit, you resist doing those things which in the first place will help you not to become overweight, and so it rapidly becomes a vicious cycle.[69]

Professor Andrew Prentice

Gluttony or sloth?

67. Determining the root causes of obesity is central to any efforts to tackling it, and, according to an influential paper published in 1995 by two of our witnesses, Susan Jebb and Andrew Prentice, scientists at the Medical Research Council Human Nutrition Research Centre, "uncertainty over the aetiology of obesity remains one of the chief barriers to designing effective strategies for prevention and treatment."[70] Although much research has been carried out into the potential influence of genetic factors, such as possible metabolic defects, these have been largely abandoned, particularly as the dramatically escalating rate of obesity documented in recent years has occurred in a relatively constant gene pool. Instead, the key question remains that articulated by Susan Jebb and Andrew Prentice in 1995:

> It is certain that obesity develops only when there is a sustained imbalance between the amount of energy consumed by a person and the amount used up in everyday life. But which side of this energy balance equation has been most altered in recent decades to produce such rapid weight gain? Should obesity be blamed on **gluttony**, **sloth**, or both?[71]

68. It is clear that people are overeating in relation to their energy needs, and that the cheapness, availability and heavy marketing of energy-dense foods makes this very easy to do, coupled with an increasing reliance on snacks and ready-prepared meals which makes selecting 'healthy' foods[72] harder. However, according to Jebb and Prentice:

---

69   Q296

70   "Obesity in Britain: gluttony or sloth?" *BMJ* 1995;311:437-439 (12 August)

71   Ibid

72   In this report we refer at times to 'healthy' and 'unhealthy' foods. Below we discuss in detail the arguments surrounding the use of these terms. We are ourselves satisfied that they are appropriate descriptions and that most experts and indeed the public at large would accept them. Unhealthy foods tend to be energy-dense, and high in fats, sugars and/or salts.

The paradox of increasing obesity in the face of decreasing food intake can only be explained if levels of energy expenditure have declined faster than energy intake, thus leading to an over-consumption of energy relative to a greatly reduced requirement.[73]

69. Summing up the energy equation, the Royal College of General Practitioners suggested that food intake had fallen on average by 750 kcal per day; but activity levels by 800 kcal. Out of this small imbalance has come the wave of obesity.[74]

Nutritional causes

Changing nutritional habits

70. Although, according to Jebb and Prentice, "it is generally assumed that ready access to highly palatable foods induces excess consumption and that obesity is caused by simple gluttony", in their view the National Food Survey in fact points to an overall drop in energy consumption since the 1970s.[75] Even after adjustments for meals eaten outside the home, and for consumption of alcohol, soft drinks and confectionery, average per capita energy intake seems to have declined by 20% since 1970. The food industry has been quick to seize upon this evidence to point the blame for spiralling rates of obesity firmly on reductions in physical activity. However, this argument ignores many other complex changes in people's nutrition patterns that have taken place in recent years, and masks the important contribution that nutrition makes to obesity. Andrew Prentice was himself displeased by this use of his research by what he termed "rogue elements of the food industry":

> We have been less than pleased at the way that paper has been wilfully misused by certain parts of the food industry, saying, "It is nothing to do with our products, it is nothing to do with food; it is all down to physical inactivity." [76]

71. An important note of warning is that the data used for the National Food Survey are self-reported, and, notoriously, individuals are reluctant to report consumption of foods they regard as being bad for them. As Tim Lobstein, for the Food Commission demonstrated:

> the latest national diet survey says [adults] are eating 82 grams of confectionery each week, self-reported. If you look at industry sales figures, those are 250 grams per week being sold to somebody. Clearly there is a huge gap between what industry is selling and what people are reporting they are eating.[77]

72. **Given the profound significance of overweight and obesity to the population we believe it is essential that the Government has access to accurate data on the actual calories the population is consuming, including figures for confectionery, soft drinks, alcohol and meals taken outside of the home. Although we acknowledge the difficulties**

---

73   "Obesity in Britain: gluttony or sloth?" *BMJ* 1995;311:437-439 (12 August)

74   Appendix 18

75   "Obesity in Britain: gluttony or sloth?" *BMJ* 1995;311:437-439 (12 August)

76   Q282

77   Q294

of obtaining accurate data, given the limitations of any self-reported survey, the current information is very weak and clearly underestimates actual calorie consumption. We recommend that work is urgently commissioned to establish a Food Survey that accurately reflects the total calorie intake of the population to supersede the flawed and partial analysis currently available. The Food Standards Agency and Scientific Advisory Committee on Nutrition should advise on this.[78]

73. Even if overall calorie consumption has fallen, there have been significant changes in the composition of people's diets. Firstly, there has been an increase in the proportion of fat in the British diet: in the 1940s, each kJ of carbohydrate in the diet was associated with 0.6 kJ of fat but in the 1990s with 0.9kJ of fat, an increase of 50%.[79] Although both carbohydrates and fats produce energy, exactly where and how people take in their energy has a crucial role in obesity.

74. During the course of this inquiry, the food industry has made constant use of the formulaic argument that 'there are no such thing as unhealthy foods, only unhealthy diets', a phrase we have also, perhaps surprisingly, heard from sports officials and Government ministers. But it is patently apparent that certain foods are hugely calorific in relation to their weight and/or their nutritional value compared to others:

Weight and calorie content of snack foods[80]

Snacks	Weight	Calories
Bag of Walkers crisps	35g	183
Snickers bar	61g	280
Apple	112 g	53

75. Besides portion size, calorie content is determined largely by fat, sugars and other refined carbohydrate content. More important than the total amount of energy (or calories) a food has is how much energy it contains in relation to its weight, that is to say its *energy density*. Put simply, energy density is a measure of a food's calories in relation to its total volume, and relates to how satiating, or filling, a food is. For example, a king size Snickers bar, which weighs 100g, has more calories than a main meal of sirloin steak served with potatoes and broccoli, which has a total weight of 400g.[81] Its high energy density means that the Snickers bar, although it is highly calorific, is not correspondingly filling, and so does not send the brain signals telling a person to stop eating in the same way that a filling main meal would. Foods that are high in energy density, and in particular high in fat, have only very weak effects on satiety —that is they do not fill you up. A Snickers bar, although it is in fact as calorific as some main meals, would typically be eaten as a snack

---

78 The Scientific Advisory Committee on Nutrition is an advisory committee of independent experts that provides advice to the Food Standards Agency and Department of Health as well as other Government Agencies and Departments. Its remit includes matters concerning nutrient content of individual foods, advice on diet and the nutritional status of people. See www.sacn.gov.uk.

79 Andrew Prentice and Susan Jebb, "Obesity in Britain: Gluttony of Sloth?", *BMJ*, 311 (1995), pp 437-39.

80 www.walkers.corpex.com; www.snickers.co.uk; www.weightlossresources.co.uk

81 Collins Calorie Counter

between meals, and a person in the habit of having a Snickers bar with their mid-afternoon cup of tea could arguably be said to be having four meals a day rather than three.

76. According to Professor Prentice, humans have evolved to have an "asymmetry of appetite control", often described as the 'thrifty genotype' theory:

> We are very good at recognising hunger—it is an evolutionary obligatory fact that we should respond to hunger very well—we are very bad at recognising satiety. Indeed, if you think it through, we are almost predesigned to lay down fat.[82]

77. While in times of uncertain food availability this asymmetry could help people survive famines, in today's environment, it is very conducive to weight gain. Professor Prentice explained that while it does not necessarily pose problems for people who are very physically active, who are generally able to control their weight successfully on their hunger drive, the reverse is true for people who are very physically inactive: "the environment is pressing on you much more food than you need and your body, physiology, is just not designed to stop it; in fact it is designed to say, 'Thank you very much, I will lay that down as fat.'"[83]

78. Professor Prentice went on to describe to us how controlled experiments demonstrated this phenomenon:

> You have experimental volunteers who you ask to eat normally but you secretly change the content of their foods—then, as soon as you add fat in and increase the energy density they overeat. It is extremely easy to replicate under any experiment: they automatically overeat. The reason they do this is they continue to eat the same bulk of food, the same amount of food, without recognising—their bodies simply do not recognise—that it has more calories, more energy in it.[84]

79. While the energy density of soft drinks, which are frequently highly calorific, needs to be considered differently from that of solid foods, recent research has demonstrated that consumption of soft drinks is likely to increase normal caloric intake—in other words, when people consume soft drinks, they do not recognise that they have taken in extra energy and compensate by reducing energy from elsewhere in their daily diet, or by expending additional energy; they simply add it on.[85] A standard 330 ml can of Coca-Cola contains 139 calories. Thus if a person were to consume a can of Coca-Cola with two meals per day, over a week that would result in an energy surplus of nearly 2,000 calories—more than a whole day's recommended calorie intake for the average woman, and about three-quarters of the recommended daily calorie intake for a man. Evidence from the British Soft Drinks Association suggests that children drink an average of 4.7 litres of soft drink per week, of which only 10% are fruit juice or water.[86]

---

82 Q287

83 Q287

84 Q288

85 Q290

86 Appendix 22; Appendix 14 (Professor John Blundell)

80. Recently, the thesis that unhealthy food may have specific addictive properties has also been explored. John Blundell, Professor of Psychobiology at the University of Leeds, has argued that while there are fundamental differences between the brain's response to food and to addictive drugs, the pleasure and the positive reinforcement people obtain from eating food could lead to the development of a compulsive element to food consumption.[87] According to Susan Jebb, this is fostered not only by the taste of food but by "the whole aura surrounding food, the marketing, the lifestyle that you buy into."[88]

81. The past 20 years have seen considerable changes not simply to what people eat and how much, but also to the ways in which they eat. Snacking, eating out, and reliance on convenience food have all increased dramatically. These changing patterns of consumption are in part a response to the far reaching social changes of the last 50 years, including a greater number of women working outside the home, longer working hours, and higher levels of disposable income. However, while these changing eating patterns may not of themselves be a problem, they can be conducive to obesity.

82. Readily available snack foods and drinks are typically very energy-dense, and are usually consumed to supplement rather than replace meals, despite their high calorie content. Between 1993–98, sales of snacks to adults more than tripled in the UK, from £173 million to £541 million.[89] As the Department pointed out in its memorandum, British people now consume an increasing number of meals outside the home, with 25% of respondents to a consumer attitudes survey saying that they regularly used some form of fast food or takeaway outlet.[90]

83. There is also increasing consumer demand for convenience food, and a growing trend towards snacking and eating on the move. The average time spent preparing a meal in 1983 was an hour, but today it has shrunk to 13 minutes.[91] In the period 1990–2000 alone, purchases of convenience foods rose by 24%.[92] According to market analysts Mintel, between 1998–2002, demand for ready meals in Britain grew by 44%, compared to 29% growth across Europe as a whole, and figures suggest that Britain is now consuming the highest number of ready meals in Europe, double the amount consumed in France, and six times that in Spain.[93]

84. Eating ready prepared snacks or meals, whether pre-packed meals which are heated up at home, or food purchased from a restaurant or fast food outlet, reduces a consumer's choice and control over what they eat. When preparing a meal from scratch, a consumer will have full control over how much fat, sugar and other ingredients are put into the dish, control over what quantity to make, and over the portion size that is served. Buying a snack such as a bag of crisps, or a ready-prepared meal to heat up, effectively removes those

---

87 Q367 (Susan Jebb)

88 Q367

89 http://news.bbc.co.uk/1/hi/business/your_money/102413.stm

90 Ev 9

91 "Can't Cook. Won't Cook. Don't Care. Going Out", *The Times,* 17 November. 2003

92 National Food Survey 2001

93 http://news.bbc.co.uk/1/hi/uk/2787329.stm

choices. People eating out in a restaurant are even less likely to be aware of the fat or calorie levels of the meal they have ordered.

85. Consumption of alcohol, particularly amongst women and young people, has increased dramatically during the past years.[94] With most alcoholic drinks being at least as calorific as a high-sugar soft drink, such as Coca-Cola, it would seem intuitive that the massive increase in their consumption has had some impact on the nation's weight. Much attention has focused in recent months on the growing culture of 'binge drinking', particularly amongst young people. While the health risks associated with this are well documented, what is less publicised is that drinking five pints of lager over an evening adds an extra 1,135 calories, nearly half a man's daily energy requirement, and five bottles of an 'alcopop' such as Bacardi Breezer contain 990 calories, nearly half a woman's daily energy requirement.[95]

86. During the course of our inquiry, we have been continuously surprised by the lack of emphasis given to the impact of alcohol consumption on obesity. While the Department, and most experts who gave evidence to us were in no doubt that it must have an impact, there seemed very little definitive evidence in this area. We were also concerned to note that the Government's recent Alcohol Strategy made no mention whatsoever of the potential impact of alcohol consumption on weight gain, leading to a further set of health problems in addition to those already linked directly to alcohol.[96]

87. **The relationship between alcohol consumption and obesity is too little understood. We recommend that the Department of Health commissions research into the correlation between trends in alcohol consumption and trends in obesity.**

Information and choice

88. What people consume is, at its simplest level, determined by personal choice. However, changing lifestyles have made the nutritional environment, spanning supermarkets selling ready meals, restaurants, sandwich bars and fast food outlets, increasingly complex, and this means that making healthy, informed choices about nutrition is more complicated than ever. The nutritional environment of the United States was described in stark terms by Marion Nestle, from the Department of Nutrition, Food Studies and Public Health, New York University, who argued that American society had changed in ways that made it "much, much too easy for people to over-eat":

> Food is extremely cheap in our country, and there are many, many driving forces keeping the cost of foods extremely low. Low-cost food encourages people to eat more. Food is extremely convenient; it is ubiquitous; it is available all day, 24 hours a day, 7 days a week; and it is available in larger and larger portions ... Every single one of those aspects encourages people to eat more, and there is a considerable amount of research that demonstrates that. We have created a societal environment in which it is considered totally acceptable for people to eat anywhere, to eat all day long and

94   Ev 8

95   http://www.weightlossresources.co.uk/calories/calorie_counting/christmas_alcohol.htm

96   *Alcohol Harm Reduction Strategy*, Cabinet Office, March 2004

to eat in larger and larger quantities; all of which encourages people to eat more and to gain more weight.[97]

89. While the UK may be some way behind the US in terms of its obesity epidemic, our evidence suggests that the information and tools consumers require to negotiate a changed nutritional environment have not kept pace with those rapid changes, and that frequently external factors are directing consumers towards unhealthy rather than healthy choices.

90. Information and education are clearly key to making healthy choices about what and how much to eat. Yet although the evidence-base about what constitutes a healthy diet has been well developed for many years, it is clear that people are not adhering to healthy eating recommendations. According to the Food Standards Agency (FSA), British children eat fewer than half the recommended portions of fruit and vegetables a day, and the vast majority have intakes of saturated fat, sugar and salt which exceed the maximum adult recommendations.[98]

91. Why, then, are these messages not getting through? Perhaps they are not being delivered loudly or consistently enough, meaning people are simply unaware of how to balance foods to make up a healthy diet that does not lead to weight gain. Alternatively, people may be insufficiently aware of the devastating health consequences associated with being overweight or obese. According to Tim Lobstein of the Food Commission healthy eating messages are well known, but external pressures prevent people from adhering to them:

> When I go and give talks to even low-income families, they are fairly well aware of the sorts of things they ought to be eating more of, but they are not doing it and they are not doing it for a variety of cultural and economic reasons—and also for children there are fashionable reasons and so on. There are a number of other pressures besides the health education message that are encouraging them away from healthy eating.[99]

92. We address these other pressures, including commercial food promotion and food pricing later in this chapter.

93. In addition to a good theoretical understanding of what constitutes a healthy diet, being able to prepare a healthy meal is a cornerstone of healthy eating habits. Yet we have received evidence suggesting that a growing number of British people lack the basic skills and confidence to do this. The Nutrition Society also argued that the "lack of ability to cook amongst the school generation means that people are not as in control of their food supply as they might be."[100] Focus on Food echoed these sentiments by stressing that dietary behaviour could not be changed without teaching people relevant skills such as cooking, which reduce the reliance on high-fat, high-salt, processed foods.[101] The need for such skills to be taught is all the more marked, given that, for the first time, the current

---

97   Q461

98   Food Standards Agency, (June 2000), *The National Diet and Nutrition Survey of Young People aged 4 to 18 years*, HMSO, London

99   Q303

100 Appendix 13

101 Appendix 34

generation of children is being raised by parents whose main experience of cooking is preparing convenience foods, thus removing a major source of food education from children.

94. The national curriculum currently includes Food Technology under the remit of Design and Technology, and this covers learning about food preparation, food hygiene and the design of food products. Food Technology is compulsory up until the age of 11, but after that there is no compulsion for any practical cooking skills or food education to be learnt. Moreover the Qualification and Curriculum Authority states that the focus of Food Technology should be on manufacturing and processing food rather than practical cooking skills.

95. The dire state of cookery provision has led to a number of initiatives where mobile facilities for cookery teaching, dubbed 'Cooking Buses', travel to schools providing lessons for children and training for teachers. The existence of these schemes has clearly tapped into an unmet need and enthusiasm for cookery training at school, as many of these schemes have waiting lists of over a year.[102]

96. Even if people are well aware of what constitutes a healthy diet, and have full information about the nutritional value of what they are eating, their decision-making does not take place in a vacuum. Any health information about nutrition that consumers currently receive is heavily counterbalanced by advertising and promotion campaigns undertaken by the food industry.

Table 5: Advertising spend across the top ten advertised food brands in the UK (2002)

	Spend (£'s)	% of Total
MCDONALDS – Fast-food restaurant	41,973,066	9.3%
COCA COLA, ORIGINAL COKE – Soft-drink	15,531,274	3.4%
KENTUCKY FRIED CHICKEN – Fast-food restaurant	15,140,219	3.3%
BURGER KING – Fast-food restaurant	11,168,498	2.5%
PIZZA HUT – Fast-food restaurant	9,357,014	2.1%
COCA COLA, DIET COKE – Soft-drink	7,395,695	1.6%
PRINGLES, CRISPS – Savoury-snack	6,700,914	1.5%
KIT-KAT, CHOCOLATE BAR – Confectionery	6,469,021	1.4%
WEETABIX – Breakfast Cereal	6,366,666	1.4%
KELLOGG'S, CORN FLAKES – Breakfast Cereal	6,263,369	1.4%
TOTAL (all food brands)*	451,956,091	

Source: A C Nielsen cited in the Hastings Report (see below) 2003

Table 6: Children's after-school snack products, market size and advertising spend, 1998–2003

	Market size 1998 £m	2002 £m	Adspend 1998 £m	2002 £m
Chocolate bars and countlines	3,745	3,494	68.9	91.0
Crisps and snacks	2,078	2,385	30.5	31.4
Sweets**	1,770	1,768	38.6	39.5
Sweet biscuits	1,484	1,462	7.2	16.3
Fresh fruit	2,962	3,150	4.5	2.8

** includes sugar confectionery and chewing gum
Source: Nielsen Media Research/Mintel

97. Figures from the Mintel study into advertising costs revealed that only a fraction of the amount of money spent advertising chocolate, sweets, crisps and snacks was devoted to advertising fruit. While a total of £178.2 million was spent in 2002 on advertising chocolate bars, crisps and snacks, sweets and sweet biscuits, over the same period only £2.8 million, less than 2% of this total, was spent on advertising fruit. Meanwhile, the £5 million annual budget of the Government's Five-a-day campaign is simply drowned out by the advertising budgets of large food companies.[103]

98. The food industry also deploys a full range of less explicit and visible, but no less effective, promotion techniques, such as inclusion within packs of collectible free gifts to encourage repeat purchase, and strategic placement of products within stores. Examples of this include placing high-sugar soft drinks in refrigerators alongside fruit juice, giving over a prominent end-of-aisle space to one product, or placing sweets near checkouts where they are guaranteed a captive audience of fractious children and hassled parents. In doing this, food manufacturers work closely with food retailers, in particular large supermarkets. While this relationship appears to work to the mutual benefit of both food manufacturers and retailers, the impact on the consumer may not be so positive. Packaging, pricing and the design of the products themselves are also used to encourage consumption. It is because product design is driven by consumer preference that so many children's food items are nutritionally poor. It was noticeable—and deeply regrettable—that when four food manufacturers (Pepsi/Walkers, McDonalds, Cadbury's and Kellogg) were giving evidence to us, only Kellogg gave a straight answer to the question "How much of your product would you advise a parent to give their five year old?" The other three representatives simply equivocated.[104] This points up the challenge facing parents when trying to help their children to eat healthily.

99. All these marketing efforts come together in evocative brands that have great emotional and psychological power. In a world increasingly dominated by such brands it is noticeable that the market leaders in the food industry—Coca Cola, McDonalds, Walkers—represent relatively unhealthy food options and are aimed heavily at children. However, the increasing availability of suitably healthy fruit and salad options at some fast food outlets is welcome if these are promoted energetically.

103 Department of Health press release, 5 October 2001

104 Qq 771, 774, 784, 786

100. While food advertising is an ever-present and accepted part of daily life, it is assumed that adults are sufficiently media-literate to be able to separate advertising claims from fact, to recognise the commercial motivation of advertising, to balance advertising messages against other relevant information, such as healthy eating messages, and to make their decisions accordingly. However, questions are now being raised about the legitimacy of explicitly targeting children, who may not be as able as adults to negotiate the pressure put on them by food advertising. According to the International Association of Consumer Food Organisations, children may be "technologically savvy" but they are "nutritionally inexperienced and ill-equipped to distinguish inflated sales messages from objective fact."[105] This is particularly concerning given that the promotion and advertising of unhealthy foods is targeted far more intensively at children than at adults: we were shocked to hear from research carried out by Sustain that during children's programming, adverts were screened between two and three times more frequently than during adult programming:

> Food advertisements were shown more frequently during children's programmes (45–58% of all advertisements) than during adult programming (21%).

> The overwhelming majority of the foods advertised during both adult (86%) and children's (**95–99%**) programmes were high in fat, sugar and/or salt.

> There were **no** adverts for fresh fruit and/or vegetables during either the adult or children's programmes.[106]

101. In addition the FSA commissioned a systematic review of the literature from a team of academics headed by Professor Gerard Hastings, at the University of Strathclyde (hereafter 'The Hastings Review'). This examined the academic literature on the amount and nature of food advertising to children over the last 30 years. It concluded that:

> children's food promotion is dominated by television advertising, and that the majority of this promotes pre-sugared breakfast cereals, confectionery, savoury snacks, soft drinks and, latterly, fast-food outlets.

102. It goes on to state that concerns should not be limited to television advertising and indeed that "There is some evidence that the dominance of television has begun to wane in recent years." The review suggests two reasons for this trend:

> First, the rise of new media (eg. computers, text-messages, internet and email) has given rise to a host of new potential creative strategies, in themselves more likely to be both accessed and understood by young people than their parents (compared to television). Secondly, the evolution of brand stretching and globalisation has allowed promotional messages to cut across many different media and increased tie-ins with below-the-line marketing activities. These may now include links to new media (eg. branded, perhaps online, computer games), other new promotional channels (eg. in-

105 International Association of Consumer Food Organisations, *Broadcasting Bad Health*, July 2003, p 8.

106 Parliamentary Office of Science and Technology, *Improving Children's Diet*, September 2003, p 45.

school marketing) and more traditional avenues for below-the-line activities such as sports sponsorship.[107]

The review went on to conclude that:

> The advertised diet varies greatly from the recommended one, and that themes of fun and fantasy or taste, rather than health and nutrition, are used to promote this to children. Meanwhile, the recommended diet gets little promotional support.

103. It is not difficult to see why children are prime targets for food industry promotion and advertising—a report in *The Observer* cited a food industry publication arguing that for soft drinks companies, an eight-year old boy was the ideal target customer, as he had 65 years of consumption ahead of him.[108] Marketers also engage in what is known as 'cradle-to-grave' marketing which is essentially relationship marketing with children. In recognition of children's potential as consumers to a firm over their lifetime, promotion can be used to create and foster ongoing relationships with them. Usually strategies of this kind focus on branding in an effort to develop an emotional and enduring connection between the child and the brand. Academic research has shown the importance of brands to children of all ages; the relationships that children form with brands often become central components of their lives.[109] Promotion is used to encourage children to develop awareness of and preferences for a particular brand.

104. Advertising agencies and food manufacturers were quick to describe today's generation of children as "media-aware" and argued that they were perfectly able to recognise advertising for what it was and interpret it accordingly from as young as five years old.[110] However, Andrew Brown, Director General of the Advertising Association and also representing the Food Advertising Unit, admitted that children did not know the full persuasive influence of advertising until they were about eight or nine, and research suggests that children below the age of five years generally regarded advertising solely as entertainment.[111] Academic research confirms that there is real cause for concern about advertising to children. Understanding of its persuasive intent only emerges at 7–8 years.[112] Prior to this, children show very little ability accurately to judge and critically to reflect upon commercial messages, and as a result are very trusting of them. One study showed that 64.8% of 6–7 year old children reported "trusting all commercials".[113] At around the age of 8 years, there is evidence that children are *beginning* to respond to advertising in a more sophisticated and critical way.[114]

---

107 Gerard Hastings et al, *Review of Research on the Effects of Food Promotion to Children*, Centre for Social Marketing, p 98

108 "The Junkfood Timebomb that threatens a generation", *The Observer*, 9 November 2003

109 M F Ji, "Children's relationships with brands: 'True Love' or 'One-Night Stand?", *Psychology and Marketing*, 19(4): 369-87; M Lindstrom, and P Seybold, *BRANDchild*, 2003

110 Q624

111 Parliamentary Office of Science and Technology, *Improving Children's Diet*, September 2003

112 D R John, "Through the eyes of a child: Children's Knowledge and Understanding of Advertising", in Macklin MC, Carlson L (eds), *Advertising to Children – Concepts and Controversies*, 1999

113 T S Robertson, J R Rossiter (1974), "Children and commercial persuasion: an attribution theory analysis", *Journal of Consumer Research*, 1974, pp 13-20

114 D R John, "Through the eyes of a child"

105. It is clear advertisers use their increasingly sophisticated knowledge of children's cognitive and social development, and careful consumer research into their motivations, values, preferences and interests, to ensure that their messages have maximum appeal.[115] Moreover, our inquiry showed that children as young as three years old are being deliberately targeted by UK food companies.

106. We used our powers to send for persons, papers and records to require the advertising agencies working for a number of popular fast food, carbonated drink, cereal and confectionery manufacturers to supply material to us. We requested the following information from Abbot Mead Vickers, concerning accounts for Pepsi-Cola and Walkers Wotsits, from Leo Burnett, concerning accounts for Kellogg's Cocopops and McDonald's, and from Coca-Cola directly: contact reports; client briefs; creative briefs; media briefs; media schedules; advertising budgets; market research reports; links to other communications; and links to marketing strategy.

107. The promotional material supplied by Leo Burnett for the McDonalds campaigns gave detailed information relating to 12 different campaigns for Happy Meals within a one-year period, targeted at different aged children, ranging from 3–11 years.[116] There is no nutritional information relating specifically to the calorific content of Happy Meals on the McDonald's UK website, but by adding the calorific content of different components, a Happy Meal with a cheeseburger and a regular coke can be shown to contain 613 calories, which could represent nearly half the daily caloric need of a six year old girl, and over half that of a three year old girl.[117] There were a total of **98** toys to collect over a period of one year—if a child were to collect all the toys they would require a Happy Meal every 3.7 days. One McDonald's campaign, Microstars, ran for a five-week period and had 20 toys to collect in the series. To collect all the characters free the child was required to average four Happy Meals per week during the promotional period, consuming 2,452 calories per week solely from Happy Meals, and a total of 12,260 calories over the five-week period. When questioned about this, Bruce Haines, for Leo Burnett, argued that toys were not designed to promote consumption, telling us that:

> the toys in a Happy Meal are considered by children to be an intrinsic part of the product, as is the packaging in which the food and toys are presented ... the toys themselves are available for purchase in a McDonald's for about 99 pence in any case, so you do not actually have to eat the food to collect them. They are not free.[118]

108. However, this was directly contradicted by the creative and client briefs for some Happy Meal campaigns, which made it clear that an aim of some promotions was to "get children to believe 'I've got to have a Happy Meal so that I can have an X toy'."[119] We were also told by McDonald's that:

---

115 H Stipp , "New ways to reach children", *American Demographics*, August 1993, pp 50-56.

116 Material relating to the various advertising campaigns cited in this report was submitted as "commercial in confidence" to the Committee. While we have quoted selected material from these campaigns, contained in an analysis produced by the Centre for Social Marketing, University of Strathclyde, at Appendix 61, we have agreed not otherwise to release commercially confidential material.

117 See Annex 3

118 Q592

119 Appendix 61

> The objective of the promotion is not principally to drive people to come in more often, it is largely designed to get different people to come in to our restaurants ... our intention is of course to raise the frequency slightly, but it is very slightly.[120]

109. Again, this was directly contradicted by the client brief, which stated that there was "scope to increase frequency from light to heavy users."[121]

110. Manufacturers and advertising agencies told us that advertising food to children could never be argued to undermine healthy eating messages, as ultimately parents retained full control over what children ate as it was they who bought their children's foods.[122] However, recent research has shown children's own spending-power to be increasing considerably. The Mintel report on snacking noted a steep rise in the average amount of pocket money allocated to children between 1997–2001. On average, 5–16 year olds enjoyed a 45% increase in their pocket money over the period, such that the average amount of weekly pocket money was £6.53.[123] The authors of the report noted that "with an average of over £6 per week to spend on themselves, children can easily afford snack foods." Crisps and savoury snacks are the most popular after-school snack for children and "this form of savoury snack is within almost all children's budgets. Indeed a number of brands specifically target children and are competitively priced at 10p or 20p."[124]

111. Furthermore, the written evidence we requested from advertising agencies revealed that despite the Advertising Standards Authority (ASA) code banning this, many campaigns have pester power as an explicit aim: the Wotsits client brief had a specific aim of getting children to "pester their parents to buy them", and in the Media Strategy Brief the stated "desired consumer response" for the campaign was "Wotsits are for me—I'm going to buy them when I get a chance and pester Mum for them when she next goes shopping." Walkers, whilst acknowledging the inappropriateness of 'pester power' as an explicit aim of the campaign, sought to downplay its significance, and cited the fact that the campaign had been passed by the ASA.[125] However, **we were appalled that a £710,000 campaign, launched by one of Britain's largest snack manufacturers, deliberately deployed a tactic which explicitly sought to undermine parental control over children's nutrition by exploiting children's natural tendency to attempt to influence their parents. The fact that this campaign was approved by the Advertising Standards Authority does not exonerate it, but merely demonstrates the ineffectiveness of current ASA standards and procedures.**

112. The food industry's most frequently rehearsed argument in relation to the impact of advertising and promotion on the consumption of unhealthy foods, and hence its potential role in obesity, was that these tools simply increased the market share of a particular brand of food or drink, rather than expanding the total market by encouraging the consumption of a particular food group, such as chocolate or sweet fizzy drinks. Similar arguments have

---

120 Q770

121 Appendix 61

122 Q594, Q763

123 Mintel report, *After school snacking* (2002) p10

124 Ibid

125 Q859

been rehearsed by the tobacco industry, as we noted in our report into that industry.[126] However, the Secretary of State for Culture, Media and Sport was clearly able to see this argument for what it was:

> *Dr Naysmith*:   I just wonder what do you believe on that when advertisers come and tell you, as they tell us, that all they are doing is trying to get a bigger share of the market for their brand when, in fact, what they are doing is trying to create a bigger market?

> *Tessa Jowell*:   I suspect in practice it is a bit of both. What they are trying to do is to get you to buy Galaxy instead of Cadbury's milk or whatever it is, but they are also trying to increase overall levels of consumption, of course I understand that.[127]

113. As well as being an obvious commercial aim of those in the food industry, it is also clear from large-scale research that advertising of foods to children does have a marked effect on the category of foods they select as well as the brand. The Hastings Review, published in September 2003, provided the clearest evidence yet that advertising had a direct impact on the category of foods children selected, and increased consumption of unhealthy foods.[128] The food industry refused to accept the findings of this report, and commissioned its own report to rebut the findings of the Hastings Review and the large body of evidence on which they were based.[129] To resolve the issue, the FSA then commissioned an independent evaluation of the Hastings Review, which fully endorsed both its methods and conclusions.[130]

114. Advertising and promotion of foods to children is not limited to television, shops and restaurants, and we were surprised to learn of the full extent of food promotion now taking place in schools. Recent initiatives by Walkers and Cadbury's, which attempted to involve schools in promotion schemes by rewarding the purchase of crisps and chocolate with sports equipment for schools, were described by Susan Jebb as "an absolute Trojan horse", although both of these received full backing from Government ministers.[131]

115. According to Kath Dalmeny of the Food Commission, school breakfast clubs, originally conceived to ensure children received a healthy breakfast before school, are increasingly having to work in conjunction with the food industry:

> Some of the breakfast clubs have sponsored foods that are given out, because the school needs to find funding for the breakfast club, so particular manufacturers will sponsor them. I have seen Burger King sponsoring some of the breakfast clubs. While it might not mean that there will be Burger King foods being supplied necessarily to the schools, the fact that branded goods—which may be high in fat,

126 Health Committee, Second Report of Session 1999-2000, *The Tobacco Industry and the Health Risks of Smoking*, HC 27 para 89

127 Q1424

128 Gerard Hastings et al, *Review of Research on the Effects of Food Promotion to Children, prepared for the Food Standards Agency – Final Report*, Centre for Social Marketing, 22 September 2003.

129 www.fau.org.uk/content/pops/brian_youngliteraturereview.pdf

130 Professor Stan Paliwoda and Ian Cranford, An analysis of the Hastings Review, "The effects of food promotion on children", December 2003, www.food.gov.uk

131 Q313

high in sugar, high in calories—are associated with those healthy eating schemes and associated with the endorsement of the school is problematic, I think, because it gives the message to children that these are good options to choose, that they are a regular part of their lives.[132]

116. An increasing number of schools also provide schoolchildren with access to unhealthy foods through vending machines installed in school premises. Schools are in many respects a 'captive market' for the food industry, as often vending machines represent the only opportunity schoolchildren have to purchase drinks and snacks during the school day. The motivation for schools to install vending machines is clear, as in total they contribute over £10 million each year to school budgets.[133] However, the impact on children's nutrition and health may be less positive. A pilot study funded by the FSA and carried out in 12 secondary schools has recently concluded that when given the option, children do make healthy choices. The 12 schools all installed vending machines containing healthier drinks, such as milk, water and fruit juice, and approximately 70,000 healthier drinks were bought during the 24-week duration of the trial.[134]

117. Supplying healthy meals at school not only provides an opportunity to influence a young person's nutritional and calorific intake in a positive way, but can also encourage young people to try new, healthy food they might not otherwise have access to, and shape their eating habits outside school. However, our evidence suggests that, far from doing this, school catering arrangements allow children to eat very unhealthily. The prevalence of cafeteria-style food outlets that allow pupils to opt out of healthy choices in favour of unhealthy ones remains high in schools, and a report by the Consumers' Association argued that the majority of school lunch menus "read like fast food menus"[135]. This is in stark contrast to the school lunch we sampled in Finland, where children were given no other option but a filling, healthy lunch, which included a portion of salad but no pudding, with the choice of beverage limited to water or milk. This confirms the findings of one of the key studies uncovered in the Hastings Review which showed that vending machines in school could be used to encourage the consumption of healthier food options with appropriate signage, pricing and offerings.[136]

118. With much school food provision now contracted out to independent suppliers, the onus appears to be on delivering palatable foods as cheaply as possible, with little recourse to health benefits. Sustain reported that some schools have available as little as 40p per child to provide the ingredients for a two course lunch.[137] The Welsh Food Alliance argued that according to one large commercial catering contractor, English public schools spend twice as much as the state sector on food ingredients for school lunches.[138]

---

132 Q380

133 Schools may receive an income of £10–15,000 per annum. See www.laca.co.uk.

134 http://www.food.gov.uk/multimedia/pdfs/vendingreport.pdf

135 Ev 391

136 S A French et al, "Pricing and promotion effects on low-fat vending snack purchases: The CHIPS Study", *American Journal of Public Health*, Vol 91, 1 (2001), pp 112-17

137 Ev 109

138 Appendix 38

119. Food labelling, detailing the calorific and nutritional content of foods, is a key element of the information people need to make healthy choices, and inadequate labelling can have a negative impact on nutrition in several ways. First, if nutritional information is absent, unclear or misleading, this could encourage the purchase of a product which a consumer would not buy if it were clearly labelled as high in fat or calories. An example frequently cited in our evidence was that of products claiming to be 'light' options when in fact they were still high in calories, and products claiming to be '70% fat free', putting the onus on consumers to notice that that this actually meant the product was 30% fat, and would in fact be termed by the FSA as containing a lot of fat.[139] Health claims may also be made on high calorie products to promote purchase, for example claims that breakfast cereals boost concentration and healthy bones, when the same health benefits could be accrued from products with a far lower calorie content.

120. Currently, nutritional labelling in England is largely voluntary. Not only does this mean that on some foods nutritional labelling can be entirely absent, but even when food is labelled, there is little consistency about the format or size of labelling, making it difficult to interpret or even to see. Some products give information per 100g, and some per packet, which is less useful for a consumer than the same information presented by serving. Even when products do give nutritional information by serving, the size of a 'portion' may vary between brands.

121. While there are many problems and inconsistencies about nutritional labelling on pre-packed food, information about the nutritional content of food purchased in restaurants or take-aways is virtually non-existent, and since this is now the fastest growing food sector, this problem is set to increase.

122. Despite the barrage of information consumers receive about food, whether through labelling, advertising, promotion, or health education, price remains a key determinant in choice, with research suggesting that cheap food is the priority for consumers using supermarkets. While 'healthy' versions of foods are becoming increasingly available, and consumers are seemingly very willing to buy them (research by the Consumers' Association suggested that 38% of shoppers claimed they would be willing to pay a little extra for foods carrying a 'healthy' logo[140]), instead of fostering this desire to eat healthily, the food industry appears to be exploiting it by selling foods with reduced fat or calories at considerably elevated prices. A recent survey by the Food Commission, illustrated that a shopping basket of 'healthier options' was 51% more expensive than a basket of standard processed foods. In April 2003, an article in *Health Which?* on supermarket healthy eating ranges, such as 'Good for You', 'Be Good to Yourself' and 'Eat Smart'[141] identified that in some cases there could be up to 200% price difference between the healthy and standard versions. In addition to this, they argued that many of the healthy options offered very little or no calorie saving, with some simply containing a smaller serving of the identical product.

123. Price differentials are likely to be even greater when healthy versions are compared to supermarkets' 'budget' lines. Most supermarkets do not offer healthy alternatives within

---

139 www.food.gov.uk

140 *Health Which?* , April 2003

141 *Health Which?*, April 2003

their own budget brands aimed at people shopping on a smaller budget. In a recent survey in the *Sunday Herald* ASDA was the only supermarket of the 'Big Five' which offered low-fat alternatives within its economy range, although it admitted that the items had "not consciously been developed as low fat".[142] In fact, research carried out by the Consumers' Association in February 2002 suggested that on average budget brand crisps had more fat, calories and saturated fat than standard versions.[143]

124. Naturally healthy foods such as fresh fruit and vegetables are also considerably more expensive than non-healthy alternatives. Comparing the prices of various fruits with high calorie snacks certainly demonstrates pricing differences. On the Tesco online shopping website, bananas are priced at approximately 13p each, with apples varying in price between 17–34p each. 'Funsize' small pears, marketed at children, cost 18p each, and satsumas are more expensive at 21p each. By contrast, small chocolate bars, some marketed specifically at children as 'breaktime' size, varied in price between 8p for a Milky Way to 16p for a Snickers. Crisps were even cheaper. Tesco's own brand crisps cost just 5p per bag for the budget range, or 8p per bag for the standard range, with Walkers branded crisps available at 11p per bag.

125. While many supermarkets claimed to support Government initiatives to promote fruit and vegetables to children, according to research carried out by Friends of the Earth pre-prepared fruit and vegetables packaged to appeal to children were being sold at vastly inflated prices by several of them. For example, Tesco's Kids Snack Pack carrots cost £5.50 per kg, 13 times the price of Tesco's 'value' carrots, while ASDA's 'Snack pack carrot crunchies' cost 10 times the price of normal carrots.[144]

126. An important form of price promotion is the phenomenon of 'super-sizing', where food is sold in larger quantities or portion sizes at little extra cost. Super-sizing is now visible everywhere from fast-food outlets, where it originated, to supermarkets. Although McDonalds have now withdrawn the largest of their super-size sizes, Julian Hilton-Johnson confirmed in evidence to us that all McDonald's staff are trained to promote super-size portions verbally when serving customers.[145] According to Professor Andrew Prentice, the falling cost of foods has directly contributed to super-sizing, as it is now very easy to use "bigger is better"[146] as a marketing tool. Susan Jebb, as a dietician, felt that super-sized portions were entirely superfluous to the energy needs of a normal person, arguing that "there is almost nobody in the UK who needs super-size portions, our energy needs are lower than ever."[147]

127. The evolution of super-size food portions began with the introduction of the McDonald's Big Mac in 1968 and accelerated in the 1970s with value meals, special packaging, promotional campaigns, and lower prices.[148] McDonald's Corporation

---

142 Mona McAlinden, "Supermarkets fail to cut fat in 'value' brands", *Sunday Herald*, 23 November 2003 (based on a survey of the five leading supermarket chains in the UK: ASDA, Safeway, Somerfield, Sainsbury's and Tesco).

143 "Do supermarkets' budget lines mean shrewd shopping or are they just a false economy?", *Health Which?*, February 2002,

144 Friends of the Earth, press release 8 November 2003, www.foe.co.uk

145 Qq 836-38

146 Q369

147 Q368

148 "The Gorge-Yourself Environment", *NY Times*, 22 July 2003

executive David Wallerstein initiated the super-size hamburgers, french fries and colas in the 1970s, taking his lead from the cinema industry, where high mark-up of jumbo-sized snacks like popcorn and cola led to higher profits.[149]

128. Food companies in the USA have been able to cut prices and spend more money on innovating new and larger food products because of the drop in prices for sugar, soybean, corn, palm oil, meat and other commodities. When food price inflation reached an all-time high in the early 1970s, consumer groups mobilised and agricultural policies were reformulated to ease regulation and increase production.[150] The price of sugar fell with the discovery of a way economically to produce a cheaper sweetener called high-fructose corn syrup (HFCS) in 1971. This invention ended years of unnaturally high sugar prices due to foreign aid policies. HFCS was six times sweeter than cane sugar and could be made from corn so the cost of production was much lower, allowing companies to produce more food for equal or less cost. Low price led both Coca-Cola and Pepsi to switch from a 50–50 blend of sugar and corn syrup to 100% HFCS, saving both companies 20% in sweetener costs.[151] From the mid–1970s American trade policies also ensured low prices for palm oil. By the early eighties the price of every single commodity was down. Meat production worldwide soared as feed costs of soy meal and corn fell. Calorie-dense foods at supermarkets were more affordable due to growing surpluses of US corn producing more HFCS.[152]

129. So why are healthy foods so expensive, while unhealthy foods are sold so cheaply by comparison? Much of our evidence implicated the European Union Common Agricultural Policy (CAP), through its subsidies for withdrawal and destruction of good quality fruit and vegetables to maintain prices, consumption aid for butter, consumption aid for high-fat milk products in schools, and subsidies to promote sales of high-fat milk products and wine.[153] According to Tim Lobstein of the Food Commission:

> Food supply is a lot of the push towards why our diets have been shifting over the last few years. The surplus amounts of sugar and butter and vegetable oils, which have been created under the Common Agricultural Policy, have to find a home somewhere. Surplus foods are disposed of and destroyed but the extra fats and oils all go into our food supplies.[154]

130. The problems with the CAP stem from the basic provisions of the original Treaty of Rome, which put the focus on trade and economic issues, with little or no concern for public health. This has to change if Britain's health is to improve.

131. Professor Marion Nestle, from the Department of Nutrition, Food Studies and Public Health, New York University, in compelling evidence to us, argued that food overproduction was the root cause of obesity in the United States, which currently

---

149 Greg Critser, *Fat Land : How Americans Became the Fattest People in the World*, 2003.

150 Ibid

151 Ibid

152 Ibid

153 For example, Alan Maryon Davies, Q567.

154 Q358

produces approximately 3,900 calories of food per day for every man, woman and child in the country, roughly double the average calorific need.[155]

132. While we have not had the scope or expertise, during the course of this inquiry, fully to explore the agricultural and economic policies behind food pricing in the UK, it is apparent that the current situation does very little to facilitate consumers making healthier nutritional choices.

Causes of obesity related to physical inactivity

133. There is little doubt that the nation as a whole is not as active as it should be. Current Department of Health advice is for individuals to undertake at least 30 minutes of moderately intensive activity (e.g. brisk walking) on at least 5 days a week. However, only around 37% of men and 25% of women currently achieve this target.[156] Levels of activity in the UK are below the European average which is part of the explanation for higher obesity rates.[157] For children and young people, the Department of Health advice is that they should undertake one hour of moderate activity each day. The Chief Medical Officer's recent report into the impact of physical activity and its relationship to health "confirms that, according to the best evidence, these recommendations remain appropriate for general health benefits across a wide range of diseases."[158]

134. *Game Plan*, the strategy for delivering the Government's sports and physical activity objectives, jointly produced by the Department for Culture, Media and Sport and the Cabinet Office Strategy Unit in December 2002 estimated the cost of physical inactivity in England at around £2 billion per year, a figure roughly equivalent to the £2.2 billion spent at that time by Government and lottery sources on sport. Each 10% increase in activity across the population has a potential gain of £500 million.[159]

Changing lifestyles

135. The NAO report *Tackling Obesity in England* stated that the extra physical activity involved in daily living 50 years ago, compared with today was the equivalent to running a marathon a week.[160] So why have lifestyles changed so dramatically in the past 50 years? A first answer lies in the increasing use of motorised transport instead of active methods of transport, such as walking and cycling. The latest National Travel Survey indicates that the average person now walks 189 miles per year, a fall of 66 miles over 25 years.[161] According to Tom Franklin, of Living Streets, it is clear that "we are walking less than we have probably ever done in history."[162] Mr Franklin attributed the decline in walking to the loss

---

155 Q461

156 Health Survey for England

157 Ev 118 (National Heart Forum)

158 Department of Health, Chief Medical Officer, *At least five a week: Evidence on the impact of physical activity and its relationship to health*, 2004, p 2

159 Ev 163 (Living Streets), *Game Plan: A Strategy for Delivering Government's sport and physical activity objectives*, p 47

160 NAO, *Tackling Obesity in England*, 2001, p 13

161 Ev 163

162 Q 489

of opportunities to walk, as well as to increased access to motorised transport. He argued that people would not walk to local services, be they schools, hospitals, GP surgeries or shops, that were sited more than 15 minutes' walk away, and moreover that increasingly services such as these were covering larger areas and so moving further away from residential centres.[163]

136. Measuring how active people are is difficult. The traditional approach has been to rely on questionnaires but such self-reporting is unreliable. As Chris Riddoch, an expert in physical activity based at Middlesex University, told us:

> People will report what they remember doing. They tend to remember the things they plan to do. If they went for a walk with the dog they will remember that. What they do not remember are all the incidental things they do like nipping up the stairs to the office on the floor above. Self-report measures have a fairly large amount of error built in to them.[164]

> A more effective measurement is achieved by the use of pedometers which record the actual number of steps taken each day.[165]

137. The increasing use of cars has led to a vicious circle of car dependency, as town planning has increasingly prioritised the needs of motorists above those of pedestrians and cyclists, meaning that in many places walking and cycling are at best unpleasant and at worst dangerous. At the same time, local neighbourhoods are increasingly perceived by parents as unsafe for children to play out in, implicitly discouraging active play and forcing children back in front of the television set. This phenomenon was repeatedly described by our witnesses.

138. England now reflects the result of two generations of planning centred on the use of cars. Car parks are readily available, but bike racks are not. Employees who want to walk or cycle to work frequently have no place to get showered and changed when they arrive at the workplace.

139. Tom Franklin suggested to us that the conditions for the pedestrian had actually deteriorated over the last half century: "The focus of people who are managing our streets has been about moving the traffic as fast and efficiently as possible and pedestrians have been shoved to one side."[166] John Grimshaw for Sustrans noted that the Highway Code stated that motorists should give way to pedestrians at junctions but that "no pedestrian who is alive has ever obeyed that rule."[167]

140. Pedestrians and cyclists are the 'second class citizens' of Britain's roads:

---

163 Ibid

164 Q 490

165 Pedometers are instruments attached to a person's waist which measure the number of steps taken. Some models will translate these into numbers of kilometres or miles walked and also calculate calories used in walking. The cheapest pedometers cost under £10.

166 Q496

167 Q499

What you find is that people walking are sent underground, they are sent over bridges, they find railings at the side of the pavement so they cannot cross where they want to cross.[168]

141. The Environment, Transport and Regional Affairs Committee (whose remit is now covered by the Office of the Deputy Prime Minister), in 2001 undertook a major inquiry into walking in towns and cities, in which they argued:

In contrast to the changes made to every town and city to ease motor transport, walking has been made ever more unpleasant. Pedestrians have been treated with contempt. We are corralled behind long lengths of guard railing, forced into dark and dangerous subways and made to endure long waits at pedestrian crossings … The short walk to the shops has been made unpleasant so that the commuter can get to the centre of town more quickly.[169]

142. Dr Nick Wareham of the Institute of Public Health, University of Cambridge, graphically illustrated the decline in cycling when he pointed out that 23 billion kilometres were cycled in the UK in 1952 but only 4 billion kilometres were now cycled annually.[170] The decline in cycling has occurred at the same time as the UK car population has grown in size. Whereas there were 16 million cars in 1975 there are 27 million today.[171]

143. Cycle use in European countries such as the Netherlands differs from Britain where cycling drops off markedly in the mid-teenage years, particularly for women, whereas Dutch men and women maintain healthy cycle use into adulthood and old age. CTC, the national cyclists' association, suggested that cycle training was a key component in maintaining use.[172]

144. Less tangible, but probably at least as pertinent, has been the reduction in physical activity in everyday life arising from mechanised tools, warmer dwellings, labour-saving devices, lifts and escalators, more sedentary jobs, and the pursuit of more sedentary leisure activities. Only 20% of men and 10% of women are employed in active occupations. Television viewing has doubled since the 1960s, when the average person watched television 13 hours a week compared to 26 hours now.[173]

Children's activity levels

145. The Chief Medical Officer's recent report into physical activity suggested that 2 in 10 boys and girls undertake less than 30 minutes activity a day.[174] Once again, changes in lifestyle must bear much of the blame for the levels of activity of young people.

---

168 Q560 (Tom Franklin)

169 Environment, Transport and Regional Affairs Committee, Eleventh Report of Session 2000-2001, *Walking in Towns and Cities*, HC 167 para 4

170 Q339

171 www.racfoundation.org; www.dft.gov.uk

172 Appendix 8

173 Appendix 18 (Royal College of General Practitioners)

174 *At least five a week*, p 9

146. According to the organisation Working for Cycling, in 1985–86 only 22% of 5–10 year olds were driven to school; that figure had risen to 39% by 1999–2000. Paul Osborne of the National Heart Forum noted that fewer than 1% of school journeys were made on bicycles in this country. That compares to about 15–20% in Germany and 50% in Denmark.[175] This may be because at least one-third of primary schools have effectively banned cycling to school by refusing to allow children to bring bicycles onto the premises.[176]

147. As Tom Franklin for Living Streets pointed out, the impact of lowered physical activity will not fall simply on the health of the present generation of schoolchildren, but will be carried into adulthood and will be perpetuated when today's children become parents themselves:

> For the first time ever less than half of our young children are walking to school. They have learned habits which they will take with them through the rest of their life which is that you drive round the corner rather than walk round the corner.[177]

148. Once at school, children struggle to meet the Government's target of two hours of PE per week. A national survey by Sport England indicates that Government guidelines on sport in schools have had mixed results. The survey showed that the percentage of children who do not take part in any sport at school on a regular basis had increased from 15% in 1994 to 18% in 2002. On the other hand, the percentage of children receiving two hours or more of PE a week increased from 33% in 1999 to 49% in 2002 (although the rate of increase seems to be slowing, with a rise of only three percentage points since 1994).[178] This last result is positive in that it shows the amount of PE in schools does seem to be increasing, although it remains a fact that one in two children does not receive at least two hours of PE in the curriculum. The Government aim therefore remains aspirational.

149. Our predecessor Committee, in its report into *Public Health* in 2001, noted that in many European countries, such as Austria, Norway, Portugal, Spain and Switzerland, an average of 3.5 hours per week was spent on school sport.[179] The European Heart Network has recommended a statutory minimum three hours per week dedicated to physical activity for all ages of young people.[180]

150. Activity levels appear to have fallen in every aspect of children's lives. Len Almond, from the British Heart Foundation National Centre for Physical Activity and Health, pointed to a "substantial decrease" in children's activity levels during school break-times, telling us that some schools had even put seats in playground so that children could sit down for the whole of the lunch break. There has also been a major reduction in active play at home, with children engaged in far less activity at weekends than they are between Monday and Friday. According to Professor Almond, active play:

---

175 Q388

176 Q396

177 Q476

178 Appendix 19 (Sport England)

179 Health Committee, Second Report of Session 2000-01, *Public Health*, HC 30, para 191

180 European Heart Network, *Children and Young People – the Importance of Physical Activity*, December 2001, p19

is simply being completely eroded (1) through lack of opportunities to play and (2) through the fact that there is no repertoire of games or activities that children can play … They have no repertoire of games or activities to play because they have lost it all, it has been lost over a number of years, and as a consequence boredom—"I'm bored"—is very often a thing that young people complain to their parents at school holidays and weekends.[181]

3 Solutions

151. In an article covering an interview with Melanie Johnson MP, Minister for Public Health, in November 2003, the *Health Service Journal* called her attitude towards the obesity issue "surprisingly sanguine" and "remarkably relaxed". The Minister described Government action on obesity as follows:

> We are doing a lot of things on obesity already—we have a food and health action plan under way. We have the Five-a-day programme, the schools fruit scheme. I'm not sure you need a strategy because we are talking about some very simple messages—take a bit more exercise, eat a bit better, make sure your children do the same.[182]

152. In direct contrast to this, obesity experts from whom we received oral evidence repeatedly stressed the complexity of the problem of obesity, and the naïvety of approaching it in such a simplistic way. Dr Susan Jebb told us "one of my key points is there is no one simple solution. If there was, we would have done it by now."[183] Professor Jane Wardle, of the Health Behaviour Unit at University College London, argued that as "it has been multiple small changes in society which have contributed to the changing population weights", "we are going to have to intervene in multiple ways to push it back down again, there is not one simple answer."[184]

153. **The causes of obesity are diverse, complex, and, in the main, underpinned by what are now entrenched societal norms. They are problems for which, as our expert witnesses have emphasised, no one simple solution exists. However, to fail to address this problem would be to condemn future generations, for the first time in over a century, to shorter life expectancies than their parents. A recent report by the Royal College of Physicians, Royal College of Paediatrics and Child Health, and the Faculty of Public Health emphasised the need for solutions to be "long term and sustainable, recognising that behaviour change is complex, difficult and takes time."[185] We believe that an integrated and wide-ranging programme of solutions must be adopted as a matter of urgency, and that the Government must show itself prepared to invest in the health of future generations by supporting measures which do not promise overnight results, but which constitute a consistent, effective and defined strategy.**

154. Recent months have seen commentators remarking with increasing frequency on the need to transform the current provision of healthcare in this country from a national illness service to a true national health service, and a White Paper positioning public health as a central plank of this Government's health policy is expected later this year. Although it may not currently be delivering all it could in terms of preventative medicine, many of our witnesses explicitly stated that this country's primary care based health service puts the UK

---

182 *Health Service Journal*, 6 November 2003, pp 26-27

183 Q315

184 Q256

185 *Storing up problems*, p xii

in a uniquely strong position to tackle obesity as a public health problem. We consider NHS provision for both prevention and treatment of obesity later in this chapter. However, **while the NHS is clearly central to tackling obesity through providing specialist health promotion and treatment for people who are already obese, we believe that the most important and dramatic changes will have to take place outside the doctor's surgery, in the wider environment in which people live their lives. And while we recognise that individuals have a key role to play in determining their own health and lifestyles, as the main factors contributing to the rapid rises in obesity seen in recent years are societal, it is critical that obesity is tackled first and foremost at a societal rather than an individual level.**

155. In his recent report *Securing Good Health for the Whole Population* Derek Wanless remarked:

> Evidence-based principles still need to be established for public health expenditure decisions. Although there is often evidence on the scientific justification for action, there is generally little evidence about the cost-effectiveness of public health and preventive policies or their practical implementation.[186]

We acknowledge that this is the case. Clearly, it is not within our resources to attempt to cost the solutions we propose in this chapter; that is a matter for Government. We are however encouraged by Mr Wanless's own observation on the need for taking action even in the absence of a comprehensive evidence base:

> The need for action is too pressing for the lack of a comprehensive evidence base to be used as an excuse for inertia. Instead, current public health policy and practice, which includes a multitude of promising initiatives, should be evaluated as a series of natural experiments.[187]

156. Obesity is a perfect example of an issue that demands truly joined-up government action, with the work of at least six separate government departments directly impacting on it. As well as the Department of Health, which retains lead responsibility for obesity as a public health issue, the Department for Culture, Media and Sport has policy responsibility for promoting sport and physical activity, and also for the media, including the advertising of foods. The Department for Education and Skills has responsibility for ensuring children receive adequate physical education at school, as well as responsibility for the food children have access to in school, and for children's education about nutrition and food preparation. The Department for Transport has responsibility for ensuring that transport policies support healthy transport such as cycling and walking; the Office of the Deputy Prime Minister has responsibility for promoting urban spaces in which people can pursue healthy travel and recreational activities; the Department for Environment, Food and Rural Affairs has an influence through its remit for farming and food production; and the Department of Trade and Industry has a stake in this debate through its responsibility for the food manufacturing and retail industries. The Department for Work and Pensions could also be influential, in that it oversees this country's increasingly sedentary working lifestyles. The

---

186 Derek Wanless, *Securing Good Health for the Population*, Final Report, February 2004, p 5

187 Ibid, p 121

list might be further widened were we to include other areas of Government on which obesity, if left to accelerate unchecked, is likely to have an impact in future years.

157. However, despite reassurances from Ministers, our evidence does not suggest that the Government is yet considering obesity in such broad terms, or even that those parts of government with a more obvious and immediate stake in the obesity issue have been working together successfully. Although Imogen Sharpe, Head of Cardiovascular Disease and Cancer Prevention at the Department of Health, told us about no fewer than seven separate boards, initiatives and meetings taking place across the Government to consider issues which might have an impact on obesity, in none of these did the issues of physical activity and diet appear to be linked together. Two Government Ministers from different departments have so far lent their approval to food marketing schemes aimed at children, whereby children are encouraged to purchase and consume high-fat foods, such as chocolate and crisps, in exchange for contributions towards school sports equipment. The Food Commission has calculated that "in order to obtain a 'free' basketball worth around £10, some £71 would need to be spent on 170 chocolate bars. A child would have to play basketball for 90 hours to expend the 40,000 calories and 2kg of fat from that amount of chocolate."[188] These initiatives were robustly condemned by the FSA, and we learnt that neither they nor the Department of Health were consulted prior to these schemes receiving ministerial endorsement, starkly revealing the contradictions that have arisen within policy concerning obesity.[189] Tim Lobstein, of the Food Commission, expressed extreme frustration with this:

> I think top of your list is going to have to be a recommendation that governments bang each other's heads together, that is to say you need a cross-departmental nutrition and physical activity policy. I talked to Tessa Jowell quite recently and she could only see the sports side of her department and would not listen to any discussion about the media side, which is advertising.[190]

158. We were very surprised that when we sought oral evidence from officials from DEFRA to discuss aspects of food production policy and its potential impact on obesity we were repeatedly rebuffed by that Department, who maintained that they had no part to play in discussions concerning obesity. Eventually, after intervention by the Secretary of State, a witness from DEFRA did appear before the Committee, but through no fault of his own had not been briefed to talk about those issues we considered most central to his Department's influence on obesity, and had no responsibility in respect of the Common Agricultural Policy. We were later supplied with written information on the Common Agricultural Policy by the Secretary of State, which is discussed below.

159. **We feel strongly that the problem of obesity needs to be recognised and tackled at the highest levels across government. We therefore recommend that a specific Cabinet public health committee is appointed, chaired by the Secretary of State for Health, and that one of its first tasks is to oversee the development of Public Service Agreement (PSA) targets relating to public health in general and obesity in particular, across all relevant government departments.**

188 Ev 109

189 Q14

190 Q357

160. Experience in Scandinavia and in other countries where dietary change was needed has shown the value of having a public health co-ordinating council or other body which operates in the public domain and maintains the drive for cross-governmental action. It can also provide a regular overview of the determinants of diet and physical activity and the effectiveness of interventions. To that end, **we recommend that the Government should consider either expanding the role of an existing body or bodies, such as the Food Standards Agency or Central Council of Physical Recreation (or linking these), or consider the creation of a new Council of Nutrition and Physical Activity to improve co-ordination and inject independent thinking into strategy.**

Nutritional solutions

161. The previous chapter discussed the causes of obesity at length. Although the debate about whether nutritional changes or physical activity changes have been the main driver of the increases in obesity is still ongoing, it is clear that to tackle obesity effectively, whether through the treatment of existing obesity or prevention of future obesity, solutions need to be found that will address both sides of society's changing energy balance: that is to say to reduce the intake of calories through altering nutritional intake, and to increase energy expenditure through changing physical activity habits.

162. As we have noted, energy intake at the beginning of the twenty-first century is very different from that of 50 years ago. While people in Britain may technically be consuming fewer calories, they are overeating in relation to their energy needs, are eating far greater proportions of fats and are having their normal appetite control overridden by the increasing availability of highly energy-dense foods and soft drinks. At the same time lifestyles have changed dramatically, meaning that people rely heavily on convenience foods. The British consume the highest number of ready meals in Europe; snacking is up; eating out is up. These trends, driven by far reaching societal changes, are not ones that it would be possible or even necessarily desirable to attempt to reverse. But there are certain tools today's population need if they are to be able successfully to negotiate what several witnesses have termed an increasingly 'obesogenic' environment.[191]

Information and choice

163. Altering people's dietary habits would appear to be an obvious and simple starting point in tackling obesity, and in their evidence, the Department put considerable emphasis on their actions to date in addressing the nutrition side of the obesity equation. They cited ongoing work on a Food and Health Action Plan, which was announced in December 2002 as part of the Government's strategy for Sustainable Farming and Food, although no date has been set for publication. The Department also drew attention to the National School Fruit Scheme, and the Five-a-day health promotion programme, both of which aim to increase consumption of fruit and vegetables.

164. However, it is clear that, as solutions to the obesity epidemic, the fruit and vegetable promotion schemes favoured by the Government have significant limitations. First, although the consumption of five portions of fresh fruit or vegetables a day is accepted as

---

being beneficial in its own right, it is difficult to see precisely how this will help tackle obesity, unless it is assumed that consuming more fruit and vegetables will displace calories from other sources. The Government's fruit and vegetable campaigns only stress the importance of consuming fruit and vegetables—they make no suggestion that these should be consumed as snacks instead of, for example, chocolate or crisps. The same holds true for the Free School Fruit scheme, which is currently only being made available to very young children aged between four and six.

165. The Government has recently invested £7.5 million on an advertising campaign aimed at stopping people smoking. By contrast, although we were told by the Public Health Minister that obesity commanded the same priority as smoking,[192] there have to date been no public health education campaigns directly aimed at reducing obesity through nutritional changes, or by any other means.

166. Research suggests that the recent anti-smoking advertising campaign has already had a small, but significant impact.[193] It is interesting to note that this campaign has relied heavily on shock tactics, employing unashamedly graphic depictions of arterial fat accumulation caused by smoking. While smoking and nutrition have obvious differences, this suggests that negative messages are capable of generating a powerful impact.

167. While we strongly endorse the Government's efforts to reduce smoking, it seems odd that so much sustained effort and investment has been put into this while no steps at all have been taken to tackle obesity, despite its occupying, according to the Public Health Minister, joint top priority with smoking. Indeed, the Government has also invested substantially in other health education campaigns on issues which, although clearly important, have not been identified by Government as a top public health priority, during the time that obesity has received none. For example, £40 million has been targeted towards reducing teenage pregnancy between 2003–06, and £4 million spent on a sexual health education campaign over two years.[194]

168. We in no way wish to imply that any of these areas of public health are undeserving of the attention and funding that the Government has invested in them. Indeed, our own recent inquiry into *Sexual Health* identified this as a very important and neglected area of public health.[195] However, what it does seem to suggest is that the Government's approach to public health education over the past few years has been responsive rather than pro-active, and has not been informed by any kind of sustained strategic prioritisation.

169. In his recent report into public health, Derek Wanless argued convincingly that since the demise of the Health Education Authority (HEA), no single body has held strategic responsibility for public health education campaigns. When we put this to the Public Health Minister she told us that the Health Development Agency was carrying on the HEA's work successfully. However, we received no evidence at all from the Health Development Agency for this inquiry into a major public health issue, a fact that we feel speaks for itself. **We strongly endorse the Wanless Report's recommendation that the**

192 Q1304; Q1306

193 http://news.bbc.co.uk/1/hi/health/3579313.stm

194 Department of Health, press release 2002/0499, 28 November 2002

195 Health Committee, Third Report of Session 2002–03, *Sexual Health*, HC 69

Government must assign clear responsibility for the health educational role, previously played by the Health Education Authority, a fact made clear in correspondence from the Department to the Committee.[196]

170. We were very surprised that despite its occupying 'joint top priority' on the Government's public health agenda, there have been no health education campaigns aimed at tackling obesity. Although we acknowledge its benefits, we do not accept the Government's view that the Five-a-day fruit and vegetable promotion campaign is either designed for, or capable of, addressing the nutritional aspects of obesity. In recent years the Government has funded health education campaigns around, amongst other things, smoking, teenage pregnancy and sexually transmitted infections. The order in which other public health issues have been addressed, and the exclusion to date of obesity from this list, make the Government's actions in this area appear haphazard rather than strategic.

171. If the Government intends seriously to address obesity through health promotion, it must adopt a health education campaign dedicated exclusively to tackling obesity, which should follow the model used in the recent anti-smoking campaign, plainly spelling out the health risks associated with being overweight or obese, and also highlighting those nutritional and lifestyle patterns which are most conducive to weight gain. It should specifically identify 'high risk' foods and drinks, and should also emphasise the fact that consuming alcoholic drinks, like any other high-calorie food or drink, can also be conducive to unhealthy weight gain. At the same time, it should highlight the importance of physical activity both in preventing obesity and reducing weight levels. Part of the campaign should emphasise the crucial links between obesity and diabetes, and between obesity and cancer (which we have heard is barely known by the public as a whole). We recommend that such a health promotion campaign should be launched as soon as possible, with the Food Standards Agency advising on the nutritional content of such promotion, and the Activity Co-ordination Team, if this remains operational, or alternatively Sport England through its links with Move4Health[197] advising on the physical activity dimension.

172. An awareness of the importance of healthy eating is useless without the practical skills to translate this knowledge into action. As well as understanding what constitutes a balanced diet, people need to know how to identify healthy foods and how to prepare them healthily, in order to reverse the increasing reliance on ready-prepared meals which require minimal cooking skills. We have heard evidence that cookery teaching has been progressively eroded by pressure to focus on other areas of the curriculum, and that, where food technology is taught, practical lessons have largely been replaced by theoretical learning about food manufacturing and marketing.[198] For many schools the only source of practical cooking lessons is through voluntarily provided initiatives such as cooking buses. The Rt Hon Margaret Hodge MP, the Minister for Children, argued that provision of food education was now better than ever:

---

196 Department of Health, Memorandum OB 8C (*not printed*)

197 Move4Health is a co-ordinating body representing interested parties seeking to tackle physical inactivity. More information can be found at www.Move4Health.org.uk.

198 Appendix 34 (Focus on Food)

In our days we were not really taught about the ingredients and the nutritional content, or otherwise, in any great detail or the impact on our health. That link between being able to cook and linking it back into the healthiness of the ingredients you choose to cook is much stronger today than it was in the past, in some ways it is better than it was.[199]

173. Mrs Hodge also felt that food education was widely available: "food technology, as it is known today, is on universal offer in every primary school and it is available in 90% of our secondary schools."[200] However, although she told us that 100,000 students take GCSE food technology per year, this only represents approximately 16% of GCSE students.[201]

174. **Understanding the importance of healthy eating is meaningless without the skills to put these messages into practice. The huge demand for initiatives such as the Focus on Food Cooking Bus is a testimony to the extremely limited opportunities for cooking and food training within schools, and also to the desire of both pupils and teachers to have access to this type of training. While we fully support these initiatives and acknowledge the good work they are doing to bring this training back within reach of school pupils, we feel that learning about how to choose and prepare healthy meals should be an integral part of every young person's education, not an optional extra delivered only periodically. This is currently not the case. We recommend that the Government takes steps to reformulate the Food Technology curriculum, so that children of all ages receive practical training in how to choose and prepare healthy food which they can put into practice in their daily lives. As well as practical cookery lessons and classroom lessons about nutrition, children should also be taught how to understand food labelling and how to distinguish food advertising and marketing from objective fact; they could put their knowledge to the test in visits to a local supermarket. Healthy Schools initiatives have demonstrated the additional value of engaging children in projects to grow their own fruit and vegetables, fostering an understanding of where foods come from as well as reinforcing their motivation to eat more healthily. This should also form part of the food curriculum in schools. In order to achieve this, steps will need to be taken to strengthen teacher training in these areas.**

175. **We recommend that delivery of the Food Technology curriculum should be rigorously inspected by Ofsted.**

176. Although it is clearly vital to educate individuals and equip them to choose healthy options, whether in the classroom or through wider health promotion campaigns, making healthy decisions can be difficult even when people are well aware of what is good for them and what is not. The Food Commission argued very strongly that:

The obesogenic environment needs to be tackled at the highest levels. It is not adequate to focus on the individual, especially the child, and expect them to exercise self-control against a stream of socially endorsed stimuli designed to encourage the consumption of excess food calories.[202]

---

199 Q1509

200 Ibid

201 Department for Education and Skills, http://www.dfes.gov.uk

202 Ev 81

177. The central tenet of this argument was in fact backed up by the Department's own written submission to our inquiry, in which they acknowledged that while many of the determinants of obesity risk were controlled by personal choice, other, wider circumstances also played a significant part:

> People's exposure to risk reflects, in part, the choices they make about how to live their lives. But these are also heavily influenced by the circumstances in which they live—people do not have equal opportunities to make healthy choices.

> Industry has a responsibility to make it easier for consumers to choose a healthy diet, remove some of the barriers that can make it difficult to do so and provide clear and consistent information about their products.[203]

178. Recent comments from the Secretary of State for Health and the Minister for Public Health imply a belief that the public must share the responsibility for their own health, rather than rely entirely on government.[204] Given this, it is perhaps not unreasonable to speculate that the forthcoming White Paper on public health may adopt an approach that gives government the responsibility for educating people about the dangers of obesity and how they might be avoided, and leaves people to make their own decisions. However, there are serious doubts about whether such an approach would be sufficient to reverse trends in obesity, underpinned as they are by the current obesogenic environment. Evidence suggests that the vast majority of people are amply aware of the importance of healthy eating, but, as Tim Lobstein for the Food Commission told us, cultural and economic pressures outweigh the healthy eating messages they receive. According to Jackie Cox, Joint Chair of TOAST (The Obesity Awareness and Solutions Trust), there is a great misunderstanding of the problem of obesity:

> It has been seen as just a food problem—so if you teach somebody how to cook a low-fat chocolate cake, they will be cured; whereas most people in this country are quite knowledgeable about whether they should have an apple or a Mars bar, and that they should walk about more and so on.[205]

179. Professor Prentice also argued that the impact of health education was limited:

> I have gone through a transformation myself of thinking that we could do it all through education and have come to the conclusion that that is not working. I am not a nanny-statist but I am a health professional and I do think we have a responsibility to look after the health of the population.[206]

180. This diagram, shown to us by Professor Pekka Puska of the Finnish Health Institute, provides a helpful illustration of the individual's challenge to live a healthy life, in the face of a rising gradient of societal pressure to live unhealthily. While ultimately individuals must meet this challenge themselves, government can play a role both by providing

203 Ev 9

204 For example, "All talk and no action on obesity", *The Guardian*, 7 May 2004

205 Q1109

206 Q312

individuals with support as they climb, and by lowering the gradient against which they are climbing.

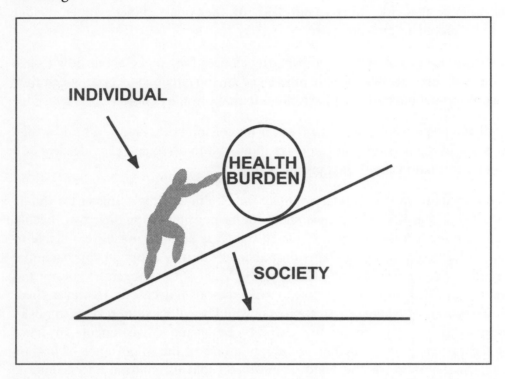

181. **Health promotion campaigns, as the recent anti-smoking advertising campaign has demonstrated, can play a successful role in raising awareness of the risks associated with particular behaviours, and to this end we have recommended that a health education campaign targeting obesity is launched as soon as possible. However, our evidence suggests that obesity has increased rapidly despite the fact that the benefits of a healthy diet have been well known for over 20 years. While we accept that individuals have the right and the responsibility to make choices about their own health and lifestyle, and we accept the importance of health education in enabling them to do so, we believe that to tackle obesity successfully education must be supported by a wider range of measures designed to remove the key barriers to choosing a healthy diet. We therefore recommend that the Government should concentrate its efforts not solely on informing choice, but also on addressing environmental factors in order to, in its own words, make healthy choices easier to make.**

Food advertising and promotion

182. While there is clearly a role for well designed and targeted health promotion schemes, one of the main doubts about their effectiveness centres on the huge financial weight of the food industry which is, by and large, directed at promoting entirely the opposite message, as articulated by Tim Lobstein of the Food Commission:

> Too much reliance has been placed on health education and handing out the odd leaflet in doctors' surgeries over the last 20 or 30 years as the Department of Health's strategy. It is not adequate. The main reason it is not adequate, of course, is that for every pound the Health Education Authority used to spend on promoting healthy diets there is about £800 being spent by the food industry encouraging us to eat their

products. Of those products, about 95% are ones that would have encouraged weight gain rather than a healthy diet.[207]

183. Particular concern has been voiced about advertising food to children, which has been shown to have a demonstrable effect not only on brands but also on the categories of foods children eat. So how far is it desirable or possible to stem the seemingly continuous stream of messages children receive promoting unhealthy foods? The solution posited by Tessa Jowell MP, Secretary of State for Culture, Media and Sport, in her evidence was that, rather than imposing restrictions or controls on the promotion of unhealthy foods, these should be countered with the promotion of healthy foods. Equally surprisingly, she went on to suggest that it should be the advertising agencies and the food industry themselves who made this investment. While we are strongly in favour of the industry being part of the solution to this problem, the Secretary of State's view struck us as rather naïve.

184. Advertising agencies are commercial businesses and cannot be expected pro-actively to fund the large-scale promotion of healthy foods for the public good. They will clearly only be able to put their 'creative genius' to good ends if they are commissioned and paid to do so, which raises the question of who might reasonably be expected to provide such funding. Government health education campaigns are one answer, but we have already seen the insignificance of Government health education budgets compared to the advertising budgets of multinational food and drink companies. Even with sustained new investment it is difficult to see that the Government would be willing or even able to match this year on year. The other option would be to rely on the food industry itself, but given that currently the fruit industry spends on advertising just 2% of the amount spent on advertising unhealthy snacks, achieving equality between healthy and unhealthy foods does not seem a realistic aim.

185. **While we would clearly support an expansion in the promotion of healthy foods to redress the balance which currently lies entirely in favour of unhealthy foods, this alone seems to be an idealistic and ill thought-through notion, one which we are surprised that the Secretary of State for Culture, Media and Sport was prepared to espouse.**

186. In the absence of this as a realistic option, the other way to redress the balance would be to impose some degree of control on the promotion of food to children. While the industry position on this is clear, this option is already under active consideration by the Government, who identified the role of regulation, particularly in relation to advertising, as an important area for consideration in the Department of Health's public health consultation, published in March 2004. The Secretary of State for Culture Media and Sport has already expressed her "scepticism" about measures targeting the advertising of food to children:

> Why am I sceptical? Well, first of all, of course I recognise the very powerful alliance that has come out today in support of a ban. Of course we will await the advice of the Food Standards Agency later this month and I will receive advice in the summer from the media regulator, OFCOM [Office of Communications], about whether or not codes that regulate food advertising on children's television are sufficiently robust. This is an extremely complex issue … The reason that I am sceptical is that

we have got to come back to the evidence. Why are we getting fatter? We are getting fatter because we are less active. [208]

187. However, the FSA has already accepted that evidence suggests that promotional activity influences children's eating habits. In the FSA's action plan, it argues that "action to address the imbalance in TV advertising of food to children is justified", and goes on to say that "action on advertising during children's TV slots would be likely to have some beneficial effect, and wider action might also be justified."[209]

188. There are recent precedents for advertising bans, both in the UK and abroad. The Co-op supermarket has already taken unilateral action in this area, by stopping all its advertising of 'unhealthy' foods and drinks during children's television programmes, as has Cadbury's.[210] Several countries have also introduced statutory regulation, or made government recommendations for strengthened voluntary controls:

- Sweden does not permit advertising aimed at children under 12, does not allow programmes to be interrupted by advertising and does not permit advertising before or after children's programmes.

- The Canadian province of Quebec prohibits all marketing aimed directly at children aged under 13.

- Norway is seeking a ban on advertisements before, during or after children's programmes.

- The Flemish region of Belgium does not permit advertising five minutes before and after programmes for children aged under 12.

- In the Netherlands the public broadcasters are not allowed to interrupt programmes aimed at under 12 year olds with advertisements.

- In Denmark, Finland and the Netherlands, characters or presenters from children's programmes cannot appear in advertisements.

- In Finland, McDonald's cannot promote toys in its advertisements.[211]

189. The Broadcasting Committee of Ireland is reported to have drafted a code whereby fast-food advertisers will be obliged to warn children that their products should only be eaten in moderation and as part of a balanced diet; advertisements for cakes, biscuits, sweets and chocolates will have to show a toothbrush symbol. Advertisements for food and drink will not be able to portray or refer to celebrities or sports stars.[212]

190. A counterargument we heard employed frequently by those who opposed restrictions on advertising food and drink to children was that no evidence yet existed that such

---

208 BBC Radio 4, The Today Programme, 3 March 2004

209 FSA Paper 04/03/02, 11 March 2004, pp 8-9, www.food.gov.uk

210 Co-op, *Blackmail*, p3

211 International Association of Consumer Food Organisations, *Broadcasting Bad Health*, July 2003, p24 and http://www.childrensprogramme.org/regulate.html

212 See www.irishhealth.com

restrictions directly yielded reductions in childhood obesity.[213] It is also the case that many children watch programmes aimed at adults such as Coronation Street, which is actually sponsored by Cadbury's (although advertising slots during such programmes are considerably more expensive). In addition, children may also be exposed to messages promoting unhealthy foods through many other media such as the internet and satellite television.

191. However, logic dictates that if advertising has an effect on the categories and quantities of foods that children eat, then removing that advertising would mean that this effect was gradually lessened, although the impact of this might not be felt immediately. Furthermore we strongly endorse the view taken by Derek Wanless that lack of evidence should not of itself be a reason for inaction.

192. **Given the scale of the public health hazard the country is confronted by, it would seem appropriate to employ a precautionary approach where evidence is contradictory. As we have said previously, we are committed to long-term solutions to the problem of obesity. The Hastings Review offered stark evidence of the extent to which advertisers of less healthy foods were saturating broadcasting slots targeting children, who are often watching without any adult present. While we would not want to go so far as to call for an outright ban of all advertising of unhealthy food, given the clear evidence we have uncovered of the cynical exploitation of pester power we would very much welcome it if the industry as a whole acted in advance of any possible statutory control, and voluntarily withdrew such advertising. There is clear evidence that the majority of parents do not favour such advertisements during children's television.**

193. **In one crucial sense, however, we share a concern about the effectiveness of banning or controlling television advertising: as noted above it is only a small part of the enormous food marketing effort that is aimed at children. If television advertising were to be banned, the marketing effort would simply be displaced to other areas— money previously spent on television advertising would, for example, be diverted to point of sale or internet promotion.**

194. **We gather that the Secretary of State for Culture, Media and Sport is in discussion with OFCOM over the marketing of less healthy foods. We would like her to review the whole marketing function. In particular, we would like her to address some of the issues the Irish Broadcasting authorities are looking at, namely the impact of product endorsement of less healthy food by sports stars, and other celebrities; guidance on how these products can actually fit into a healthy diet, perhaps linking into nutritional information; and their impact on the energy equation in terms of the activity needed to displace the calories they add. Assuming the food and advertising industry is genuine in its desire to be part of the solution, a starting point for this would be for companies to agree clear public health targets.**

195. **As we noted earlier, we were disturbed at the ineffectiveness of the Advertising Standards Authority, which is an industry self-regulation system. We recommend that OFCOM be asked to review the role of the ASA with a view to improving its**

---

213 See, for example, Q864.

effectiveness. This is not the first occasion on which the Health Committee has found the performance of the ASA to be disappointing.[214]

196. Children are subject to an onslaught of food promotion in many aspects of their daily lives, and the school environment appears to be no exception, with sponsorship by food companies and vending machines selling only unhealthy products now commonplace. When we put this to Margaret Hodge, the Minister for Children, she replied simply that this was a matter for individual schools and headteachers:

> I think it would be wrong for us in the DfES or for us in Government to prescribe from the centre what individual schools should do in relation to where they seek sponsorship. What we have done is to give guidance to say that they should measure the advantages and make sure that the educational advantages gained from a particular form of sponsorship outweigh the disadvantages and that has to be a decision for them … the individual headteacher ought to decide himself or herself what vending machines to have or what other form of promotion he or she chooses to have within their institution, and weigh up the economic and educational benefits against the disbenefits.[215]

197. However, there seems to us no logic at all in assuming that children in some areas might 'benefit' from exposure to such commercial pressures while others would be harmed. This is surely an area crying out for central guidance and direction.

198. Margaret Hodge went on to suggest that the impact of school was limited compared to the messages children received at home, arguing that "the greatest influence on children and the outcomes they achieve is the quality of parenting in the home" and that her priority would lie in "seeing how we can better support parents". However, we believe that the school is a crucial environment in which messages about nutrition—whether healthy or unhealthy—can be learnt and reinforced, sometimes resulting in children introducing to their parents healthier eating patterns learnt at school. Indeed, this is a central tenet of the Government's free school fruit campaign. We have also received evidence suggesting that children respond positively to the availability of healthy options. Where they have been trialled, vending machines selling only healthy foods have yielded a high turnover.[216]

199. **We feel that the school environment can have a strong influence over children's developing nutritional habits, and that the Government must not neglect this crucial opportunity to promote healthy eating to children and help them develop sound lifelong habits. Healthy eating messages learnt through the national curriculum and Government healthy eating initiatives such as the schools fruit campaign will be contradicted and undermined if, within that same school environment, children are exposed to sponsorship messages from unhealthy food manufacturers, and given access to vending machines selling unhealthy products. There is evidence that parents are keen to see unhealthy influences removed from schools, with recent research finding that as many as 70% of parents were in favour of banning vending machines in**

---

214 See eg Health Committee, Fourth Report of Session 2000–01, *The Provision of Information by the Government Relating to the Safety of Breast Implants*, HC 308, para 31.

215 Q1487; Q1493

216 Food Standards Agency, *A feasibility study into healthier drinks vending in schools*, Health Education Trust, March 2004, www.food.gov.uk.

schools.[217] Recent research by the FSA also indicates that children are willing to purchase healthier drinks from vending machines when they are given the option. Given the worryingly steep rise in levels of childhood obesity, we feel that parents, teachers and school governors must all be fully engaged in tackling it, and that obesity should command a high priority on school board agendas.

200. We therefore recommend that all schools should be required to develop school nutrition policies, in conjunction with parents and children, with the particular aim of combating obesity, but also of improving nutrition more generally. In conjunction with this, the Government should issue guidance to all schools strongly recommending that that they do not accept sponsorship from manufacturers associated with unhealthy foods or install vending machines selling unhealthy foods. If Government insists that this is a matter for local determination, we believe that governors should permit such practices only if these are shown to be supported by a clear majority of parents. The guidance should also give firm support for the replacement of existing vending machines with ones selling healthy foods and drinks.

Food labelling

201. Food labelling is a tool that could potentially enable consumers to choose healthier foods and negotiate their way through today's 'obesogenic society' more successfully. However, current labelling appears to fall far short of this aim. To begin with, the absence of legislation in this area means that nutritional labelling is often entirely absent from foods, and where it is present, is often complex, difficult to interpret, and in illegibly small print. Nutritional information panels are often overloaded with information, much of which may be irrelevant to the needs of today's consumers. For example, Dr Mike Rayner, Director of the British Heart Foundation, Health Promotion Research Group, argued that although when the 'Big 8'[218] standard nutrition label was devised protein deficiency was still a problem for some people in this country, almost no-one suffers from this problem any more, making the inclusion of protein on nutrition labels largely redundant.[219]

202. As well as the absence, inconsistency and irrelevance of information, the crux of the problem lies in the intelligibility of nutritional information on food labels. Sue Davies, for the Consumers' Association, told us that:

> Part of the problem is that even if you had the most comprehensive nutrition information, it is very difficult—and I have difficulty, as a consumer—to know how much fat I am supposed to have and what is a high amount of salt or a high amount of sugar. When people are shopping in a hurry, they do not want to be doing all of those calculations in their head, do they?[220]

203. Dr Mike Rayner told us that "everybody agrees that the nutritional labelling panel is completely incomprehensible, and people cannot make sense of the numbers, and there are

217 'Ban Junk Food from Schools, says poll', The Guardian, 22 October 2003

218 The 'Big 8' are defined as: energy, protein, carbohydrate with declaration of sugars, fat with declaration of saturates, dietary fibre, and sodium.

219 Q1166

220 Q1151

too many numbers."[221] According to the Consumers' Association, research suggested that consumers liked to see simple, bold claims such as 'low fat' on products, because it helped them make decisions when shopping in a hurry, without having to negotiate the nutrition panel.[222]

204. However, a problem frequently brought to our attention during the course of this inquiry was the impact of misleading nutrition claims, when products marketed as healthy failed to live up to that claim. We heard numerous examples, often relating to the fat content of foods, and in particular we were struck by the example of the cereal Frosties Turbos, advanced in evidence from the Consumers' Association. Using a series of eye-catching symbols on the front of the packet, Kellogg's claim that Frosties Turbos are good for bones, good for concentration, good for heart health and low in fat. What is not mentioned is that they are made up of 40% sugar, and that other, less sugary breakfast cereals might provide similar benefits with fewer calories.[223]

205. Andrew Coslett, for Cadbury Schweppes, argued compellingly that "an average supermarket can carry about 20,000 lines, and to try to get mum to understand every one of those in making a balanced diet is a challenge."[224] Besides improving the consistency and transparency of nutrition claims, our evidence suggested that consumers also need a simplified system of nutritional labelling for choosing foods to make up a balanced diet. The difficulty consumers may have in researching and understanding the calorie content in different foods is perhaps reflected by the fact that commercial weight management programmes often provide their customers with far simpler alternative systems for making nutritional decisions, such as the Weight Watchers Points system. However, devising a universal food classification system such as this goes to the heart of the argument surrounding whether or not any foods can reasonably be deemed 'good foods' or 'bad foods', 'healthy foods' or 'unhealthy foods'.

206. Food manufacturers have attempted to draw a clear distinction between food and tobacco, arguing that while there is no such thing as a safe cigarette, there is no such thing as a food which, seen in isolation, is dangerous:

> I think health warnings are for dangerous things. Whilst we recognise the problem I do not think that a Curly Wurly is a dangerous thing.[225]

207. This argument has been expanded and repeated by almost all those working in or concerned with the food industry presenting evidence to us, namely that there is no such thing as a healthy or unhealthy food, only healthy and unhealthy diets.[226] This was also the view expressed by the Secretary of State for Culture Media and Sport, and Sue Campbell, Chairman of UK Sport and Chief Executive of the Youth Sport Trust.[227] However, Dr Mike Rayner told us that in his opinion this myth was beginning to be broken down, ironically

---

221 Q1148

222 Q1143

223 Q1153

224 Q791

225 Q897 (Andrew Coslett)

226 Q726, Q738, Q920

227 Q535

by the very actions of government and industry. Citing schemes by government and industry to promote fruit and vegetable consumption, he argued that:

> If we are going to eat more of good foods like fruit and vegetables, then surely we have to eat less of some bad foods like confectionery, fizzy drinks and so forth? The labelling of good food … is quite often used by the industry anyway. They quite often have "healthy eating" ranges, so they are quite content to have this notion of good food. However, again, if we are going to be eating healthy foods, then there must be, conversely, just on a logical basis, some bad foods out there.[228]

208. The Public Health Minister also accepted this point:

> *Mr Burstow*: Do you accept that some foods can be classified as junk foods?

> *Miss Johnson*: I think we would all, in common parlance, accept that there are some foods that would be regarded as junk foods … I think we all know what sort of food stuffs are being referred to, broadly speaking. It is true, of course, that a small amount of any of these foods or these foods taken in on an irregular basis will not particularly harm you in themselves. It is the degree of frequency and the size of portions that is the issue.[229]

209. Sue Davis, for the Consumers' Association, supported this view:

> We have got to get over this issue about "there is no such thing as 'good' food and 'bad' food." There are definitely foods we need to be eating less of and foods we need to be eating more of, and it needs to be made clear on the front of the pack.[230]

210. Our witnesses were clear about the need for an integrated system, on the front of food packaging, to enable consumers to make an overall judgement about the food they were about to purchase. However, they did not feel that the extreme measures feared by the food industry, such as putting health warnings on high energy density foods, or labelling them with a skull and crossbones, were either reasonable or necessary. They felt strongly that food labelling and classification did not need to be pejorative, and Dr Mike Rayner instead suggested the possibility of introducing a symbol to demarcate "fun foods" or "treat foods", highlighting the need to eat them sparingly rather than regularly.[231] As Sue Davies argued, the point of such a system would be "to highlight the good, bad or in-between foods. It is not saying 'do not eat this food', it is saying 'do not consume it very often; do not eat it all the time.'"[232]

211. We also heard the suggestion that in order to link calorie consumption to energy output, food labelling could include a requirement to state how much exercise would be

---

228 Q1170

229 Q1386

230 Q1168

231 Q1179

232 Q1168

required to burn off the calories in a particular product—for example, a Mars bar would require four miles of walking for an adult.[233]

212. In Sweden, a simple system is already in place to enable consumers to identify foods that are lower in fat and higher in fibre. Under the Swedish 'Keyhole' system, a green keyhole symbol appears on the front of foods that are lower in fat or high in fibre, although it is not included on produce which is naturally lean or high in fibre, such as lean meat and fruit and vegetables. The symbol appears on, amongst other things, low-fat sausages, cheese, ready-meals and fibre-rich breads. Products must meet strict criteria about the proportion of fat, sugar and dietary fibre they contain before they are able to use the symbol.[234]

213. The FSA told us that they believed that the law relating to food labelling needed to be reviewed and changed.[235] These changes, in their view, should include making the provision of nutritional labelling compulsory.[236] They also supported a 'high/medium/low' format of labelling as the approach that worked the best with consumers, and agreed with the concept of nutritional signposting on the front of food packaging.[237]

214. **Nutritional labelling is intended to help consumers make sound nutritional decisions when buying food, but the current state of such labelling seems to be having, if anything, the opposite effect. We have repeatedly heard the argument, both from the food industry and from the Government, that there are no such things as good or bad foods, only good or bad diets. However, both the food industry and the Government have embraced the concept of labelling certain foods as 'healthy' with great enthusiasm, inviting the obvious conclusion that other foods must be, by definition, less healthy.**

215. Dr Mike Rayner told us that the Co-op had improved the nutritional panelling on foods and now used the categories "high" "medium" and "low" on the panel, a measure which we strongly commend.[238] Indeed, the Co-op's labelling as a whole struck us as exemplary in comparison with what most supermarkets managed. Dr Rayner also suggested that a voluntary scheme to improve labelling was only likely to be effective if all the major supermarkets agreed on a common scheme.[239]

216. **The Government must accept the clear fact that some foods, which are extremely energy-dense, should only be eaten in moderation by most people, and we therefore recommend that it introduces legislation to effect a 'traffic light' system for labelling foods, either 'red—high', 'amber—medium' or 'green—low' according to criteria devised by the Food Standards Agency, which should be based on energy density. This would apply to all foods. Not only will such a system make it far easier for consumers to make easy choices, but it will also act as an incentive for the food industry to re-**

---

233 Q1179

234 Swedish National Food Administration, http://www.slv.se/engdefault.asp

235 Q1258

236 Q1259

237 Q1273

238 Q1148

239 Q1160

examine the content of their foods, to see if, for example, they could reduce fat or sugar to move their product from the 'high' category into the 'medium' category.

217. **Bearing in mind Derek Wanless's suggestion that greater effort needs to be made to measure the effectiveness of different interventions, we believe that this recommendation would lend itself well to objective assessment. If the scheme we propose is accepted, it would be relatively simple to measure the impact on the range of relatively healthy and unhealthy foods offered by supermarkets, and any shift in the patterns of consumption from relatively unhealthy to relatively healthy products.**

Food composition

218. It is indisputable that high energy density foods have a particularly pronounced impact on weight gain. The Department stated in its memorandum that the *NHS Plan* included commitments to initiatives with the food industry to improve the overall balance of diet including salt, fat and sugar in food, working with the FSA. However, the Department's memorandum does not suggest that this has been pursued as a high priority or that significant progress has been made:

> Discussions with the food industry and retailers are underway on reducing the level of salt in processed foods. These discussions have demonstrated that industry have made some steps towards reducing salt in processed foods but there is scope for further action. The situation is likely to be similar for fat and added sugars. Options for working with industry on these areas will be considered through 2003–04.[240]

219. Describing the progress made so far in this area in oral evidence, Imogen Sharpe, for the Department, told us that liaising with industry to reduce salt levels, which contribute to high blood pressure although not to obesity, had been tackled as a priority over and above fat and sugar levels under specific instructions from the Chief Medical Officer.

220. The Rt Hon Alan Milburn MP, the previous Secretary of State for Health, has recently issued forthright demands for the Government to tackle food composition as a priority:

> Specifically an ultimatum needs to be placed before the industry that unless it voluntarily cuts fat, sugar and salt in food within a specified time frame then tough regulatory action will be taken to ensure that it does.[241]

221. While lowering the fat content of foods would seem a sensible aim, Professor Andrew Prentice pointed out to us that this would not achieve the objective of reducing obesity if, as he believed was already happening, food manufacturers substituted fat with other highly energy-dense foods, such as refined carbohydrates and sugars, in order to keep selling the products to people who had acquired a taste for energy-dense foods.[242] Professor Prentice argued compellingly that it was energy density that needed to be targeted rather than just fat.

---

240 Ev 18

241 "From sick care to health care: meeting the challenge of chronic disease", speech to Oxford Vision 2020 Conference, 3 December 2003

242 Q291

222. We note the Government has made efforts to date to reduce salt levels in foods, but we feel that urgent attention should also be given towards tackling obesity. We recommend that, rather than targeting sugar and fat separately, the Government should focus on reducing the overall energy density of foods, and should work with the Food Standards Agency to develop stringent targets for reformulation of foods to reduce energy density within a short time frame. While we expect that reformulation could be achieved through voluntary arrangements with industry, and while we believe that the introduction of legislation in respect of labelling will encourage industry to make the entire product range healthier, the Government must be prepared, in the last resort, to underpin this with tougher measures in the near future if voluntary measures fail.

Food pricing

223. Research has shown price to be a key factor in people's food choices, and our evidence suggests that particularly for lower income families economic concerns may override any health information.[243] Changing food prices to influence people's decision-making in favour of healthier foods could be achieved in two ways—either by increasing the prices of unhealthy foods to act as a disincentive for consumers to purchase them, or by introducing measures to lower the prices of healthy foods, making them affordable to all. In evidence to us, the Department was reluctant to discuss these issues, arguing that "obviously, it is not for government to tell industry how much they charge for a particular food." However, they did state that the forthcoming Food and Health Action plan would be considering food production, supply and availability, and within that equality of access to food.[244]

224. Opinions vary widely on the issue of introducing fiscal measures to raise the prices of high energy density or fatty foods. According to media reports, a paper prepared by the Downing Street Strategy Unit argued that the extension of VAT for some dairy produce, fast food and sweet foods would act as "a signal to producers as well as consumers and serve more broadly as a signal to society that nutritional content in food is important."[245] A report in the British Medical Journal also claimed that a fat tax could prevent 1,000 premature deaths from heart disease alone every year in the UK.[246]

225. However, critics of the idea contend that, as with any 'vice tax', rather than changing their behaviour people simply divert spending from other necessities. It has been suggested that a fat tax would disproportionately affect lower income families, who already spend a higher proportion of their income on food and drink. The plans have also attracted criticism for ideological reasons: according to Martin Paterson, of the Food and Drink Federation, "Consumers will rightly feel patronised by 'top-down' messages based on the idea that they can't think for themselves and need to be taxed into weight-loss."[247]

243 Q303; FSA Survey, 2001

244 Q127

245 "Government unit urges fat tax", BBC online news, 19 February 2004

246 T Marshall "Exploring a fiscal food policy: the case of diet and ischaemic heart disease", British Medical Journal 320 (2000), pp 301-304

247 http://news.bbc.co.uk/1/hi/health/3502053.stm

226. Value Added Tax is already levied on certain 'treat foods': savoury snacks, ice cream, confectionery and fizzy drinks (including zero calories diet drinks) all incur VAT at 17.5%. PepsiCo pointed out in their written memorandum that this has given rise to an anomalous situation, in that other, similar treat foods are zero rated, such as cakes, cake bars, plain biscuits, Jaffa cakes, cookies, Bourbon biscuits and Ginger Bread Men with chocolate eyes—but the addition of chocolate buttons on to any of these products would result in VAT being levied.[248]

227. The healthcare costs of obesity rehearsed earlier illustrate how the NHS and society have to pay for causes out of their control. The price of cheap, fatty, sugary foods, for instance, does not include the healthcare costs that may follow much later from excess consumption. In formal economic terms, when consumers purchase cheap calories, there may be further indirect costs much later. This raises complex issues which the Wanless Reports have begun to address. The recent World Health Organisation draft strategy on diet and physical activity suggested that member states consider taxes and other fiscal measures to send more health-enhancing price signals to consumers.[249]

228. **The notion of taxing unhealthy foods is fraught with ideological and economic complexities, and at this stage we have not seen evidence that taking such a significant and difficult step would necessarily have the hoped-for effect of reducing obesity. We recommend, instead, that the Government should keep an open mind on this issue, and monitor closely the effect of fat taxes introduced in other countries. We also recommend that the Government should take steps to address the anomalies in the current arrangements for VAT on unhealthy 'treat' foods as it is clearly ludicrous that VAT is levied on ice cream and fizzy drinks but not on Bourbon biscuits or cakes.**

229. The other side of the food pricing equation would be to attempt to lower the prices of healthy foods so that they present a realistic and affordable alternative for everyone, as currently healthy foods, both 'healthy' versions of pre-prepared foods, and naturally healthy fruit and vegetables, can cost significantly more than non-healthy alternatives.

230. **We hope that as the Government and food industry work together to reduce the energy density of foods, the need for 'healthy' options will be gradually reduced, with standard versions of foods being healthy as a matter of course. However, as this is likely to be a phased process, we recommend that in the short term the Government must work with the food industry to ensure that 'healthy' versions of foods, with reduced calories and fat, are available at an affordable price.**

231. Evidence suggests that there may be considerable scope for trimming the profits attached to fresh fruit and vegetables, as according to Friends of the Earth, fruit and vegetables are significantly cheaper in street markets than in supermarkets.[250] DEFRA put average 'farm gate' prices (what a grower actually takes, after paying the costs necessary to supply the supermarket, including grading, packaging and transport) for Cox apples in

248 Ev 230

249 WHO, Global Strategy on diet, physical activity and health A57/9, 17 April 2004

250 www.foe.co.uk

October 2002 at £0.33 per kilo, while the average supermarket retail price for the same period was £1.45 per kilo.[251]

232. This inquiry has not probed in depth the complexities of European agricultural policies. However, it is clear that while the potential for the CAP to work in concert with public health policy has been recognised for over 20 years, numerous attempts to reform the CAP to these ends have failed. The UK's Committee on the Medical Aspects of Food Policy recommended that the Government should review the CAP's impact on diet as long ago as 1984, arguing that "consideration should be given to ways and means of removing from the Common Agricultural Policy those elements of it which may discourage individuals and families from implementing the recommendations for dietary change."[252] More recently, in 1999 and in 2002, this has been raised by the World Health Organisation:

> Despite a call for public health to be considered in all EU policies in 1999, no review of the CAP objectives has occurred and public health is still not mentioned as a policy determinant in the Agenda 2000 reform or in the recent mid-term review of CAP.[253]

233. According to the Consumers' Association report on the CAP, "nutrition considerations have been given scant concern by agricultural policy makers, even though diet and health are closely linked."[254] The initial reluctance of DEFRA to contribute to our inquiry on obesity could be regarded as further evidence of this continuing lack of linkage between agricultural and health policy, and the fact that the Department of Health was the last government department to respond to the Curry Commission consultation on the future of food and farming could also be seen to indicate a lack of pro-active communication in this area.

234. When a representative of DEFRA, Mr Callton Young, did eventually give evidence to us, he stated that he had not come briefed to talk about the Common Agricultural Policy. However, he confirmed that:

> The CAP does have a role to play … in terms of the health and nutrition agenda. The price of food is very clearly linked to what people buy and the extent to which it is subsidised must have a feedback down the chain to the consumer.[255]

235. Mr Young agreed that the promotion of healthier food "has to be a part of the Common Agricultural Policy."[256] However, although he emphasised the need for government departments to "look at these things holistically", when asked why his Department had not mentioned nutrition on its website he argued that that was because "the lead policy responsibilities for nutrition and health reside with the Department of Health."[257] Mr Young said that the issue of the CAP had been raised at cross-governmental

---

251 Ibid

252 "Setting aside the CAP – the future for food production", Consumers' Association, 2001, p 13

253 WHO global strategy on diet, physical activity and health: European regional consultation meeting report, p. 11, Copenhagen, Denmark, 2-4 April 2003.

254 "Setting aside the CAP", p 48

255 Q1195

256 Q1196

257 Q1201

steering group meetings for the Food and Health Action Plan, but he feared that what could actually be done about the CAP was "a much more difficult nut to crack".[258]

236. Following on from our oral evidence session, DEFRA submitted written information on the CAP, in which they told us their policy objective was to "move away from a position where the market and demand have been distorted by over-supply of some products and measures to address that over-supply." This meant, in their view, that "to this extent we will be neutralising the CAP as a force which may have contributed to increasing obesity." However, DEFRA ended on a note of pessimism, stressing the need to be realistic about what reform of the CAP could and could not achieve, and arguing that "in reality the CAP is not a particularly important factor in causing obesity."[259] This attempt by DEFRA to distance agricultural policy from health by playing down its impact does not strike us as particularly helpful in achieving joined-up solutions to this problem across government.

237. **As a matter of urgency, the Government must redouble its efforts to reform the Common Agricultural Policy as part of the public health agenda, and the future UK presidency from July 2005 will afford an opportunity for this to be done. Obesity is, after all, a growing problem in almost all EU countries. The issue of agricultural policy presents a perfect opportunity for the Government to demonstrate that it is committed to tackling public health issues in a joined-up way, an opportunity which in our view it has to date entirely neglected. However, as noted above, progress on the CAP will be extremely difficult unless public heath is given much greater emphasis in Europe. We therefore call on the Government to use its influence, and its forthcoming presidency, to encourage the Commission to reconsider the Treaty of Rome and put public health on an equal footing with trade and economics.**

238. **In the interim, the Government, led by the Treasury should emulate the Swedish Government[260] and produce a Health Audit of the CAP, and build a stronger alliance of Health Ministries to combat other interests protecting the status quo in public policy.**

239. As well as healthy food being generally more expensive than less healthy alternatives, this inequity is compounded by the now widespread use of price promotions which are heavily biased in favour of unhealthy foods. This is now an accepted part of food marketing, ranging from 'buy one get one free' price promotions in supermarkets, to super-sizing of meals in fast food restaurants and 'meal deals' on take away lunchtime foods.

240. We note that there have been improvements overall in the numbers of supermarkets where there is no confectionery available at the till. We were interested to hear that ASDA, who came out worst in a Food Commission report into this area, were now trialling the sale of fruit and non-food items at the till. We look forward with interest to hearing how this trial has gone.[261]

---

258 Q1206

259 Appendix 59

260 L S Elinde et al (2003), *Public health aspects of the EU Common Agricultural Policy*, Stockholm: National Institute of Public Health

261 Q977

241. During this inquiry we have heard repeatedly that industry is keen to be 'part of the solution'. If this desire is to be translated into reality, then supermarkets should adopt new pro-active pricing strategies that positively support healthy eating, rather than acquiesce in the view that their duty to their customers goes no further than simply providing the range of foods which they want to buy. As part of their healthy pricing strategies, supermarkets must commit themselves to phasing out price promotions that favour unhealthy foods, and also stop all forms of product placement which give undue emphasis to unhealthy foods, in particular the placement of confectionery and snacks at supermarket checkouts. Alongside this, all sectors of the food industry should collaborate in the phasing out of super-sized food portions. We expect that the food industry will be keen to capitalise on the significant commercial opportunity that introducing these policies will present, and indeed much good work has already been done in this area. Several supermarkets have already committed themselves to banning the placement of confectionery at checkouts, and Kraft and McDonalds have begun to limit the availability of super-size portions. We commend fast-food outlets for offering fruit and salad options, though we request that these should be promoted more effectively than at present. Those companies who do not comply with Government guidance on healthy pricing, including product placement and super-sizing, should be publicly named and shamed.

Food in schools

242. Throughout our inquiry, the diet of children and young people has been a recurring theme. A survey conducted by the Consumers' Association in March 2003 asked 246 children to compile a food diary which revealed that, despite the fact that children seemed to know what foods were healthy and to understand the health implications of poor diet, children in Year 6 and the girls in Year 10 ate just two portions of fruit and vegetables per day with boys in Year 10 eating just 1.5 portions. Most children ate at least one bag of crisps a day, and many had sweets or chocolate every day.[262]

243. We have already discussed in detail the promotion of unhealthy foods to children in schools, through a wide variety of schemes embraced for the commercial benefit they bring to schools without consideration of their wider health implications. In our view these should be stopped immediately. We have also made recommendations to improve the teaching of cookery in schools to teach children to choose and prepare healthy meals. However, to support improvements in both of these areas, a good example needs to be set in the school meals provided by schools themselves, something that does not seem, at present, to be happening. Again, we cannot accept that this is a matter purely for local determination by schools. Children's nutritional requirements do not vary according to where they happen to go to school.

244. In the course of our inquiry we examined the standards for school lunches that have been adopted in England and Scotland. Technically, both Scotland's standards and England's guidance include the nutrient recommendations for school meals developed by Caroline Walker Trust Nutritional Guidelines for School Meals.[263] However, the placement

262 Ev 391

263 *Scottish Nutrient Standards*, Section 1.2 and Section 1, tables 1 and 2; England Primary School Guidance, Annex Cii; England Secondary School Guidance, Annex Cii

of the nutrient guidelines within Scotland's standards and England's guidance is telling. The nutrient requirements are located in the first section of Scotland's standards which emphasise that their achievement is "essential."[264] Moreover the overall tone is that compliance is required, or at least expected; the standards speak in terms of "should," "required," and "achievement," as well as stating maximums and minimums. To this end, the Scottish Executive has commissioned the development of nutritional analysis software to assist schools in self-evaluating the compliance with these standards.[265] Caterers will be able to utilise the software to analyse the nutritional content of recipes.

245. In contrast, we were disappointed to learn that England's guidance specifically and conspicuously states that only the regulations, which do not require any specific nutrient content, are compulsory and that the guidance on good practice is "not required by law."[266] The nutrient recommendations are placed in the back of the guidelines as an annex, where it is suggested, but not required, that an approximate nutritional analysis could be accomplished by the caterer, the school food committee using a computer software package, or by an independent expert such as a community dietician.[267] The overall effect of placing the nutrient recommendations at the end, pointing out that the guidance is not compulsory, and using terms such as "aim" and "try," is that the specific nutrient content of school meals is marginal.

246. We also learned that in Scotland, standards bar the provision of fizzy drinks as a part of a school meal in primary schools, and bar the encouragement of the provision of such drinks in secondary schools.[268] Crisps, as a part of a combination meal option/meal deal or packed lunch may only be offered twice per week.[269] Neither England's regulations nor guidelines bar, limit, or discourage the provision of crisps or fizzy drinks.

247. We were please to learn from the Minister for Children that the DfES has asked the FSA and Ofsted to conduct a review of the implementation of the nutritional standards for school lunches introduced in July 2000.[270] However, we were disappointed to learn that the scope of the review did not extend to include school breakfasts.[271]

248. **We recommend that the Department for Education and Skills extend the scope of the FSA review of the implementation of nutritional standards, with a view to developing appropriate nutrient based standards for school breakfasts.**

249. **Furthermore, we recommend that the Department for Education and Skills takes steps to ensure that all children eat a healthy school meal at lunchtime, both through improving the provision of attractive and palatable 'healthy' options, and through restricting the availability of unhealthy foods. The Government should shift from the current 'food-based' standards towards the 'nutrition-based' standards being**

264 *Scottish Nutrient Standards*, Section 1.5

265 *Scottish Nutrient Standards*, Section 1.4

266 England Guidance, Section 4

267 England Primary and Secondary Guidance, Annex Cii

268 *Scottish Nutrient Standards*, Section 2, "Menu Planning" table, Group 5

269 *Scottish Nutrient Standards*, Section 2, "Menu Planning" table, Group 5

270 Q1497

271 Q1501

introduced in Scotland. The quality of school meals should also be taken into account by Ofsted inspections.

Causes of obesity relating to physical inactivity: solutions

250. Making society as a whole more active is an extremely difficult task. As we have seen, the forces promoting sedentary behaviour have grown substantially over the last few decades. There are few grounds for optimism that there will be a reversal in these trends. More and more labour-saving devices are being created, car ownership continues to grow, traffic volumes continue to increase, local shops are being replaced with out-of-town stores, and fear of crime keeps people increasingly indoors. It will require a remarkable cultural shift if society is to become more active across all social classes; a trickle of pilot projects and local schemes will not be adequate.

251. The costs to the NHS of low levels of physical activity are high. Yet as Barry Gardiner MP pointed out to us, spending on treatment dwarfs spending on promotion of physical activity, which, if adequately tackled, could offset some of those considerable health costs:

> We spend £886 per head of population per year in providing what amounts to a national sickness service and we spend £1 per person per year on sports and physical activity which could actually prevent a lot of that sickness.[272]

252. As we have noted, the current Government target for physical activity for adults is 30 minutes of moderate activity 5 times per week. Yet currently only 32% of adults achieve this, less than a third of the population, compared to 70% in Finland. The lead department on physical activity is the Department for Culture, Media and Sport. In its document *Game Plan*, jointly produced with the Prime Minister's Strategy Unit in December 2002, DCMS set a very ambitious target that 70% of people in England should attain the current activity goal by 2020. As Sport England commented, "This presents the Government—and key partners—with an exacting challenge. To put it bluntly, 100,000 inactive people will have to be converted to physical activity every single month for the next 17 years if the Government's targets are to be met."[273]

253. In this section of our report we want to examine what is being done to boost activity levels. In doing this it is important to distinguish between two separate ways in which activity is achieved:

- *organised and recreational activity, in the form of sports and other activities either in schools or in the community; and*

- *activity within daily life, which embraces areas such as active travel and activity within the workplace.*

254. These areas are not, however, entirely discrete. For example, children walking or cycling to school are likely to be fitter than those who journey by car; they are more likely to enjoy and benefit from sport; and the sporting habits they develop at school are then more likely to feed into an active lifestyle when they attain adulthood.

---

272 Q1028

273 Appendix 19

Organised and recreational activity

255. It is by no means clear that countries with high levels of active recreation and sport will necessarily be less obese—Australia has some of the fastest growing levels of childhood obesity. It may be that boosting the facilities for active recreation will in fact exaggerate health inequalities since the middle classes are much better at accessing these. The Chief Medical Officer's recent report on activity and health emphasises that physical inactivity is not merely a critical factor in obesity but also is implicated in 20 other diseases and conditions and in particular hugely increases the risk of cardio-vascular disease, diabetes and cancer.[274] In the treatment of obesity, disease reduction is just as important as weight loss and the Chief Medical Officer also supported the notion that activity significantly reduces disease in the obese.

256. The impact of school-based activities is also complex. While there is no doubt that active children tend to be less overweight and indeed to achieve more academically, organised school sport seems to alienate many children, and there is ample evidence to suggest that much bullying begins in the changing room. But while school sport occupies only a tiny fraction of the child's waking hours—around 1% a year—it perhaps is most useful in fostering habits of activity which can last a life time.

257. *Game Plan* records that levels of participation in sport have not increased much in England in recent years. Only 46% of the population take part in sport more than 12 times a year compared to 80% in Finland.[275] Following a recommendation contained in *Game Plan*, Sport England, the body charged with the strategic lead for sport, working with relevant stakeholders, is developing a national database which will provide a comprehensive audit of community sports facilities. This database will provide guidance to Government Departments, Lottery Distributors and local authorities on needs-based strategic investment priorities. The database will also provide information for the public on what facilities exist and where they are located.

258. Sport England has been modernised following *Game Plan's* publication so that its objectives now explicitly acknowledge the significance of the health agenda and its responsibility to help promote active and healthy lifestyles.

259. Many different initiatives support sport in the community but in the longer term the uptake of sport will, we believe, be driven more by what is achieved with younger people than with adults. Most of our evidence on sport and PE has focused on young people. As Sue Campbell, for the Youth Sport Trust, remarked:

> There is no question now that young people are far more sedentary by nature almost and we are creating young people who are very computer-literate, who are very engaged with other forms of learning and have almost forgotten how to learn physically.[276]

---

274 *At least five a week*, p 9

275 However, a European Commission Survey conducted in December 2002, which relied on self-reported evidence, placed the UK roughly in the middle of EU countries for physical activity. See europa.eu.int.

276 Q492

72

260. In 1999, the then Secretary of State for Education, the Rt Hon David Blunkett MP, announced his intention to address declining physical activity in schools. The National Healthy Schools Standard encouraged schools to provide pupils with a minimum of two hours of physical activity within and outside the national curriculum. However, there is no method of compelling schools to meet this standard and obese children often continue to opt out of activities outside the main curriculum. The Child Growth Foundation was moved to describe "the continued absence of any National Curriculum amendment to provide every child with the two hours per week of enjoyable structured physical activity to which they are entitled" as a prime illustration of Whitehall's inability to tackle obesity. [277]

261. In October 2002, the Prime Minister announced an investment of £459 million to deliver "a national strategy for PE, school sport and club links."[278] Both the Department for Culture, Media and Sport and the Department for Education and Skills now have a PSA target that 75% of school children should undertake two hours of high quality PE and school sport each week by 2006, and a number of programmes have been put in place to support this. The Qualification and Curriculum Authority is also exploring ways of improving PE and sport in schools.

262. To help achieve the two hours weekly target, the Government is developing School Sport Partnerships.[279] These are families of schools that come together to enhance sports opportunities for all. The partnerships comprise: a specialist sports college, eight secondary schools and 45 primary or special schools clustered around the secondaries and the College. Each partnership receives a grant of up to £270,000 each year. This funds: a full time Partnership Development Manager, the release of one teacher from each secondary school for two days a week to allow them to take on the role of School Sport Coordinator, the release of one teacher from each primary or special school for 12 days a year to allow them to become Link Teachers; and Specialist Link Teachers who fill the gaps created by teacher release.

263. Six strategic objectives have been set for partnerships:

- Strategic planning—to develop and implement a PE/sport strategy.

- Primary liaison—to develop links, particularly between Key Stages 2 and 3.

- Out of school hours—to provide enhanced opportunities for all pupils.

- School to community—to increase participation in community sport.

- Coaching and leadership—to provide opportunities in leadership, coaching and officiating for senior pupils, teachers and other adults.

- Raising standards—to raise standards of pupils' achievement.

264. By 2006, there will be 400 partnerships including 75% of schools in England. A recent survey conducted for DCMS indicated considerable success for the scheme:

277 Appendix 24

278 Appendix 44 (DfES)

279 See DfES website at www.dfes.gov.uk.

68% of pupils in schools that have been in a partnership for three years, are spending at least two hours each week on high quality PE and school sport in and after school, rising to 90% at Key Stage 3. This compares to 52% for schools new to the programme.[280]

265. The Government has checked the trend established in the 1980s of local authorities selling off school playing fields to raise capital. Active protection (through legislation introduced in 1998) and strict planning regulations has resulted in an average of only three applications a month being approved, and almost half of these are at schools which are closed or closing. In all cases, any proceeds are being ploughed back into improving sports or educational facilities—the proceeds are not being spent on school books or teachers' salaries.

266. Some £581 million is being invested in England by the New Opportunities Fund with the aim of improving and increasing sports facilities at schools. This funding will be used to support projects designed to bring about a step-change in the provision of sporting facilities for young people and for the wider community, through the modernisation and development of existing and new facilities for school and community use (including outdoor adventure facilities), and the provision of initial revenue funding in support of these developments.

267. An investment of £130 million is being allocated to 65 Local Education Authorities through the Space for Sport and the Arts programme to develop new sports and arts facilities on primary school sites. As well as benefiting schools themselves, these premises will also be available for community use, with the emphasis on inclusion of currently under-represented groups.

268. **We commend the wide range of measures and substantial funding being directed by the Government towards physical activity, particularly in schools. While we have reservations about the effectiveness of measures taken to date, we wish to pay tribute to the efforts that have been made in the last two years and to acknowledge the substantial funding that has been provided.**

269. As we noted above, the majority of children still fail to achieve two hours per week of structured activity. In many cases, schools do not have the resources to provide the suggested amounts. A House of Commons Committee of Public Accounts report found that "achievement of children's entitlement of two hours of physical exercise a week requires an adequate and equitable distribution of facilities. There is, however, a considerable disparity in the opportunities for sport currently being offered to children by different schools."[281]

270. A large amount of anecdotal evidence—including accounts given to the Committee at the 'Watch It' clinic in Leeds—suggests that obese children are often bullied, a problem that may become more acute when children are involved in traditionally competitive school sports. Many children opt out of school sports as they find competitive team sports unattractive. The National Curriculum for Key Stage 2 states that PE should be taught

---

280 See DCMS website at dcms.gov.uk.

281 Committee of Public Accounts, Ninth Report of Session 2001-02, *Tackling Obesity in England*, HC 421, p 7

through dance activities, games activities, gymnastic activities and two activity areas from swimming, athletics and outdoor and adventurous activities, although there are no specifications within these areas, and no guidelines about how vigorous these activities should be. Guidance from the DfES also stresses that provision should encourage children to enjoy PE and be keen to get involved. It is clear then that schools need to offer a range of activities in order to attract all pupils. This, however, can be difficult when resources are stretched and facilities are inadequate.

271. Barry Gardiner MP, who gave evidence to us, has proposed a more radical plan which will be piloted in four schools in Brent North from September 2004, starting with pupils in Year 7. Here, the school day will be extended to run from 8:30am–6pm, which will allow the possibility of two guaranteed hours of sport in each school day. Mr Gardiner argued that as well as improving the health of school children, the scheme would provide a number of other indirect benefits such as a reduction in youth crime, improved scholastic achievement and increased social cohesion.

272. If playing sport is not possible for some children, Mr Gardiner proposes that music, art or drama could be taught instead, which would also help relieve pressure on teaching staff. To avoid children being put off sport for life they should instead be offered "a smorgasbord, a whole range of physical activities." This might range from "ethnic dance right through to boxercise."[282] Teachers for the PE session could be assisted by volunteers and School Sports Co-ordinators (a scheme organised by Sport England).

273. Mr Gardiner's scheme also recognises the need for healthy food in schools. His proposal provides children with healthy balanced meals—an optional breakfast club in the mornings, a nutritionally balanced lunch at 1pm followed by the two hours of sport from 2pm–4pm. There would follow another break which would incorporate a carbohydrate-based snack to keep the pupils going for the rest of the day.[283]

274. A project co-ordinator will supervise the Brent scheme and £150,000 is being devoted to evaluate it. According to Mr Gardiner, initial reaction from both teachers and parents has been enthusiastic.[284] However, the response from the Government so far had, in Mr Gardiner's words, been limited to "a great many kind words".[285]

275. **We regard it as lamentable that the majority of the nation's youth are still not receiving two hours of sport and physical activity per week. While we very much welcome the DCMS/DfES target to have 75% of school children thus active by 2006 we do not believe that this goes far enough. We have reservations about the quality of much of the activity undertaken, since little work has been done to establish what the two hours involves, and whether it includes, for example, time taken in travelling to and from facilities. Moreover, even the two hour target puts England below the EU average in terms of physical activity in school, despite the fact that childhood obesity is accelerating more quickly here than elsewhere.**

---

282 Q1022

283 Ev 300

284 Q1025

285 Q1033

276. **We recommend that, given the threat of obesity to the current generation of children and taking account of the proven contribution of physical activity to academic achievement, the aspiration should be for school children to participate in three hours per week of physical activity, as recommended by the European Heart Network.**

277. **Relentless pressure on the curriculum has served to squeeze out school sport and PE. However, there is ample evidence that being physically active benefits children's academic performance, and many schools in the independent sector offer four or more hours of exercise per week. We know that the Government is monitoring closely the Brent project but that it has been less than forthcoming with supportive funding. We believe that this is a fascinating pilot project and would like to see it rigorously evaluated. Given its potential importance as a model, we also think it would be helpful if the Department's favourable initial appraisal of the scheme were supported by funding.**

278. **We recommend that the Curriculum Authority should address ways of diversifying organised and recreational activity in schools to embrace areas such as dance or aerobics to broaden the appeal of PE and to counteract the elitism, embarrassment and bullying that the changing room sometimes creates.**

279. **We do not think it appropriate that the activity of a school in delivering the physical activity agenda should be extrinsic to any evaluation of its overall performance. Physical activity is not—or should not be—a second order consideration. Not only is it crucial to children's health but it also directly benefits academic performance. So we recommend that the Ofsted inspection criteria should be extended to include a school's performance in encouraging and sustaining physical activity.**

280. The psychosocial aspects of obesity, which are often ignored in the drive to improve physical health, are particularly important in children. Obese children are frequently bullied and school sport can prove a humiliating experience. **We recommend that the Department for Education and Skills, as part of its wider work to improve self-esteem and self-confidence amongst school children, should ensure that each school, as part of its policy against bullying, remains alert to the particular issue of bullying of children who are overweight or obese. Teachers should receive training in children's diet, physical activity levels, and how to help obese children combat bullying, without further stigmatising them.**

Active lifestyles

281. When physical activity is mentioned, what springs to mind most readily is probably what Susan Jebb termed "programmed, planned exercise", such as joining a local sports team, going to an aerobics class, or using an exercise bike. However, as Living Streets argued, "for many people, joining a gym or taking part in a team sport are not realistic options—for economic or time reasons."[286] Our witnesses stressed repeatedly that rather than promoting planned sport or active recreation, which might require life changes that were unsustainable, a far more useful and realistic aim was to increase activity levels within

people's daily lives. Of these lifestyle changes, perhaps the single most important concerns transport.

282. In a report published in 1997, the British Medical Association confirmed the links between transport and health.[287] Evidence from the United States and Australia has also indicated that promoting walking can change lifestyles and improve health.[288] Many commentators have argued that a national transport plan could provide a useful tool to promote and facilitate active methods of transport. According to Living Streets, "regular walking as part of a daily routine is a viable option and involves only modest changes to lifestyle."[289]

283. Targets to increase walking and cycling within the fabric of everyday life have been set by successive governments but have totally failed. Levels of each activity have dropped to an extent which we find startling. As we have noted, levels of walking and cycling have fallen dramatically in recent years.

284. Published research from Bristol University and elsewhere using accurate measures of children's movement indicates clearly that most energy expenditure takes place when children walk to school, play out at break times and again after school.[290] Informal play seems to be more important than formal activity at least up until the teen years. Furthermore, this work shows that children are less active at weekends and in school holidays, indicating how important the school and its schedule of activities, not just formal PE and sport are to facilitating children's activity. **We believe that providing safe routes to school for walking and cycling, adequate and safe play areas in and out of school is very important in the battle against obesity.**

285. The Environment, Transport and Regional Affairs Committee in its report on *Walking in Towns* made a wide-ranging and cogently argued series of 25 recommendations.[291] These included:

- The Government should set targets to increase the level of walking.

- The Government should publish a national walking strategy.

- Planning procedures should give priority to walking.

- Conditions for the pedestrian should be improved by ensuring that walking routes are continuous, well-connected to key destinations and well-signed, and that where such routes meet major roads in urban areas, pedestrians have priority.

- Particular emphasis should be given to creating good routes to important facilities, including schools and rail and bus stations and bus stops.

---

287 BMA Board of Science and Education, *Road Transport and Health*

288 Ev 164 (Living Streets)

289 Ev 163

290 A C Cooper, et al, "Commuting to school: Are children who walk more physically active?", *American Journal of Preventative Medicine*, vol 25,4 (2003), pp 273-76 and K R Fox "Childhood obesity and the role of physical activity", *Journal of the Royal Society for the Promotion of Health* 124 (2004), pp 34-39.

291 Environment, Transport and Regional Affairs Committee, Eleventh Report of Session 2000-2001, *Walking in Towns and Cities*, HC 167, Summary of Recommendations

- More traffic-calming and traffic restraining measures should be introduced.

286. Our witnesses echoed many of these points. Tom Franklin for Living Streets suggested that there should be a pedestrian pavement run-off at every junction.[292] John Grimshaw, for SUSTRANS, gave the example of Hull to illustrate the dramatic impact of reducing traffic speeds in cities to 20 mph.[293] Hull has implemented over 100 zones with 20 mph speed limits and the total number of road crashes in the zones has been reduced by 56%. Crashes involving child pedestrians have been cut by 70%.[294]

287. **The measures proposed by the Environment, Transport and Regional Affairs Committee in its report *Walking in Towns* 2001 strike us as sensible and persuasive and we are sorry so little action has been taken to implement them.**

288. **Given the profound impact increased levels of activity would have on the nation's health, quite aside from the obvious environmental benefits, it seems to us entirely unacceptable that successive governments have been so remiss in effectively promoting active travel.**

289. The Department for Transport again suggested to us that it was aiming to publish a consultation for a national walking strategy this year. The Department for Transport set out an overarching transport strategy in its *10 Year Transport Plan* published in 2000. This put forward no targets to stop the deterioration of footways, which acts as a barrier to walking.

290. Tom Franklin for Living Streets had no doubt that the reluctance to introduce the strategy stemmed from political squeamishness:

> The problem is that the Government is almost embarrassed about promoting walking. I have to say that I think that this comes from the John Cleese sketch 25 years ago of the Ministry of Silly Walks. Since 1996 every Transport Minister has promised a national walking strategy and every one has failed to deliver … They have not delivered because each time they get cold feet because they think they are going to be perceived as the Minister for Silly Walks.[295]

291. The Department for Transport representative giving evidence to us was tentative about progress, telling us that a document would be forthcoming imminently, but that rather than a strategy this would be a consultative 'document' containing some proposals.[296] The Department organised a series of seminars, then announced a consultation in the document *On the Move by Foot*. That paper, which is extremely slight, encloses a separate report prepared by Transport 2000, not by the Department. The consultation closed in September 2003 but as yet no strategy has been put in place.

292. **We regard the failure of the Department for Transport to produce a National Walking Strategy over a period of almost ten years as scandalous. This very inactivity**

---

292 Q499

293 Q499

294 www.transport2000.org.uk/news

295 Q503; the 'Silly Walks 'sketch was actually broadcast on 15 September 1970.

296 Qq144-48

clearly demonstrates that the priorities of the Department lie elsewhere. We would be extremely disappointed if concerns about political embarrassment had indeed obstructed such an important policy. One way of defusing any political embarrassment would be to incorporate the walking strategy into a wider anti-obesity strategy.

293. Assessing the precise contribution that walking can make to combating obesity is difficult, but we have been greatly struck by the potential of pedometers to increase awareness of sedentary behaviour and thus promote activity. The Department of Health is working in partnership with the Countryside Agency and the British Heart foundation to part-fund a targeted pilot project which will distribute pedometers to PCTs in areas of high deprivation as a motivational tool to encourage increased walking. This builds on the Countryside Agency's Walking the Way to Health initiative.[297]

294. Pedometers, which are small and inexpensive electronic devices used to count the number of steps a person takes in a day, can be a very useful tool for encouraging people to live more actively. According to Tom Franklin, "people only have to wear them for a week or so before they start to get a pattern of their exercise and they start to consider, if they did that slightly differently, what the effect would be."[298] The promotion of walking plays a key part in America's strategy to combat obesity, the America on the Move initiative being piloted in the Colorado on the Move scheme.

295. Launched in October 2002, Colorado on the Move is a state-wide initiative aimed at combating obesity.[299] It has programmes to increase physical activity in schools, worksites and communities. Pedometers are distributed to help participants monitor and increase physical activity. The aim is for participants to increase their daily walking by 2,000 steps per day. It is interesting to note that, so relentless has been the rise in obesity in the USA, the goal of Colorado on the Move is not to *reduce* the weight of the population but rather merely to *stop the weight gain*. The programme is now being modified to include dietary advice.

296. So far, over 75,000 people have participated in the scheme, ranging from public sector employees, to private companies, churches and native American Indian tribes. In two pilot projects based in communities with high-risk populations in Colorado, average increases of 2,000 steps have been achieved. Within schools, children are being encouraged to make use of the pedometer data within other lessons, for example by marking the total steps taken on a map and seeing how far they have travelled.

297. In America we ourselves were given Coca-Cola pedometers, and Colorado on the Move has sponsorship from a variety of commercial sources including Pepsi. We were told that Kellogg's was considering issuing pedometers.[300] McDonalds has also very recently announced a plan to distribute pedometers with Happy Meals in 2004 in England.[301] We believe that there is great potential for pedometers in making people more aware of their

---

297 Ev 15

298 Q503

299 Information in this section is sourced from Colorado Department of Public Health and Environment, *Colorado Physical Activity and Nutrition State Plan 2010.*

300 Q877

301 *The Daily Telegraph*, 23 April 2004

general activity levels and giving them an incentive to increase these. However, the mere issue of pedometers is unlikely to do much to address the problem. People need to be told how to use them, know what targets are desirable, and learn to make increased activity a life-time habit rather than a temporary goal. **We believe it would be helpful if commercial firms issuing pedometers also issued guidance agreed with Sport England and the FSA, on the recommended activity levels per day and on the correlation between steps taken and calories consumed.**

298. If bought in bulk, simple pedometers are very inexpensive and we can envisage a range of possible providers. These could include:

- Schools, who could keep sets of pedometers for use with different classes at different times. As in Colorado, pedometer data could be incorporated into other areas of the curriculum besides PE.

- Employers, who could issue pedometers to their staff, possibly even offering incentives for their use.

- GP practices, who could offer targeted advice to individuals, and use pedometers to help address the causes rather than the consequences of obesity which is what they largely treat now.

299. **We welcome the funding the Department of Health has provided to a pilot project on the use of pedometers. We recommend that the Department co-ordinates inter-departmental activity with a view to achieving wide-spread use of pedometers in schools, the workplace and the wider community.**

300. A number of witnesses pointed to the contribution they believed that cycling could make in combating obesity. The English Regions Cycling Development Team argued that there was a suppressed demand for cycling as there are more than 20 million bicycles in the UK, many of which were rarely used.[302] Sustrans suggested that countries which were broadly socio-economically similar to the UK but with much higher cycling rates had lower levels of obesity, as this graphic demonstrates:

302 Appendix 60

Figure 1: Correlations between levels of cycling and prevalence of overweight in selected European countries

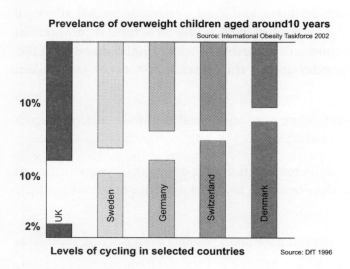

Prevelance of overweight children aged around10 years
Source: International Obesity Taskforce 2002

Levels of cycling in selected countries   Source: DfT 1996

Source: Sustrans, Ev 162

301. They contended that obesity was a symptom of the way the physical environment was planned and argued that changes should be made to encourage and facilitate active forms of travel, such as higher parking charges and improved cycling routes. In a survey of users of their National Cycle Network, 70% stated that the existence of the route had helped to increase their level of physical activity. Many of the proposals put forward by Sustrans could also link with attempts to improve healthy routes to school.[303] The Office of the Deputy Prime Minister therefore has a role to play in encouraging or demanding that town planning guidance includes measures to encourage physical activity.

302. The Department for Transport published a National Cycling Strategy in July 1996 with the target of increasing the number of cycle journeys four-fold by 2012. As part of the strategy a leaflet was published offering guidance to employers on ways to encourage their employees to cycle to work. It also referred to the co-ordination role that local authorities could play in stimulating changes to make cycling an attractive means of travel to work for more people.

303. The leaflet suggests a number of measures that employees could take to encourage cycling to work, including the provision of safe, secure and covered cycle parking, lockers, changing/drying facilities and showers and the offer of interest-free loans to purchase bicycles. The Department for Transport also pointed out the benefits to employers of this policy. By having a fitter, healthier workforce, employees will take fewer sick days and will have improved levels of concentration.[304]

304. The *10 Year Transport Plan* was published in 2000. This included an ambitious target to treble the number of cycling trips between 2000 and 2010. It provided additional funding to make conditions easier and safer for pedestrians and cyclists. The *Plan* requires authorities to prove, through Local Transport Plan (LTP) Annual Progress Reports, that

303 Ev 161

304 Department for Transport, *Cycling to Work*, 2001

they are developing and implementing strategies to secure significant increases in cycling and walking. Over the five-year period of the first LTPs, local authorities estimate they will deliver over 5,500 km of new or improved cycle tracks and cycle lanes. Around 1,200 km of cycle tracks and lanes were laid by local authorities in 2001-02 an increase of 43% on the previous year. In the same five-year period LTPs estimate that they will deliver over 1,000 km of new or improved footways and pedestrianisation schemes.

305. In 2002 two initiatives were launched by the Department for Transport to help deliver increased levels of cycling. A National Cycling Strategy Board was set up to co-ordinate and monitor implementation of the National Cycling Strategy, supported by a network of regional advisers to promote good practice and provide support to local authorities. Additionally, a Cycling Projects Fund, with £2 million funding was launched in March 2002 to support projects that can achieve a significant increase in cycling locally, or raise public awareness of the increase in cycling opportunities.

306. However, in the progress report on the ten-year plan, *Delivering Better Transport* (December 2002), only two of the 150 pages are devoted to progress in encouraging cycling and walking. This report also admits that latest available data from the National Travel Survey suggest that, as of 2001, the long-term decline in cycling and walking had not been reversed.

307. In 2002, the then Transport, Local Government and the Regions Committee expressed "little confidence" that the target for cycling increases would be met, detecting few signs of any growth in cycling in the first two years of the period.[305]

308. CTC, the National Cyclists Association, suggested some additional policies that would be useful to increase the number of cyclists, such as integrating cycling with public transport by creating cycle carriages on trains and buses, providing cycle hire facilities and doing more to tackle the growth of traffic and reduce the need to travel.[306]

309. Countries such as the Netherlands and those in Scandinavia have seen a much slower increase in obesity rates in the last 20 years and this is generally attributed to those countries' inhabitants having a much more active lifestyle, and in particular greater opportunities for active transport. In countries where there have been steady increases in cycling, such as in Denmark, there has been a reduction in casualty rates per mile. This has been achieved by "adopting comprehensive measures to create better conditions for cycling and because the more cyclists that there are, the more motorists are aware of cyclists and consequently the better they are at dealing with them."[307]

310. Again, a Health Committee report is not the appropriate forum to discuss the detailed measures required to increase cycle use on a massive scale. We can, however, record some of the key points that our witnesses made. John Grimshaw for Sustrans suggested that "Mostly any cycle lane stops exactly where you want it, at the junction." He urged that pedestrianised city centres should be permeable to cyclists. He also suggested that greater priority should be accorded to cyclists, for example by making one way streets two way for

305 Transport, Local Government and Regions Committee, Eight Report of Session 2001-02, *10 Year Plan for Transport*, HC 558, para 104

306 Appendix 8

307 Appendix 60

cyclists, as was common on the Continent.[308] Employers could play their part by ensuring that there were adequate cycle parking facilities and showers and changing rooms available.

311. Denmark is a country with some of the highest cycling rates in Europe, and cyclists are given much more priority in transport planning. We visited Odense, Denmark's third largest city, which has a population of 200,000. The Danish Department for Transport has nominated Odense as Denmark's "national cycling city." Cycle use rates are extremely high. In Odense we met local urban planners to see what made the city so appealing for cyclists.

312. It was immediately obvious that cyclists were granted a far higher status in this city than in any in England. Dedicated cycle paths, screened from cars and pedestrians, allowed cyclists access to all of the city centre. A covered cycle parking space with room for 400 cycles had replaced a car park which had accommodated eight cars. It was even possible, for a small fee, for people to lock a cycle and any valuables away in a secure automated garage facility. As in all Denmark, there is a presumption that liability for an accident involving a motorist and a cyclist lies with the motorist. This is not the case in English law.

313. The sophisticated and comprehensive cycle network we witnessed had not been designed into Odense—this is an historic city, with a cluttered centre made up of eighteenth- and nineteenth-century buildings. It has had to be integrated within an existing city, as would be the case with major towns and cities in England. We were told that the current configuration for cycling was actually the third phase of planning. For almost 20 years Odense has been working to develop cycling. We were particularly impressed to see how children were involved in the planning process. Each year, children in schools are asked to use a computer program to map their journey to school. On this, they mark any hot-spots where they feel in danger. This information is then collated and planning authorities give priority to improving conditions at these danger spots. We also commend the approach we saw in Odense, where funding support for school transport was based on the degree of danger in covering the route from home to school by other means. This provides a financial incentive on the authorities to create safer walking and cycling routes.

314. We are pleased to note that the Department of Health has recently been involved in active travel plans. According to one of our witnesses, it was essential that the Department should have an input into transport policy; for this witness at least, that had not always been the case:

> The Department for Transport has this target of increasing cycling four-fold to eight per cent of all journeys, which would more or less be in common with what was achieved in Sweden. I am sure that the Department of Health have not put their weight behind that; they probably do not even know it exists. Yet a four-fold increase in cycling would probably be more valuable for their aspirations than for the Department for Transport which is actually only interested in reducing congestion.[309]

---

308 Q502; 509

309 Q563 (John Grimshaw)

315. The Department for Transport has recently announced that it will provide funding for "sustainable travel towns". It has set aside £10 million to help develop plans for sustainable transportation in three towns in England. These towns will "incorporate all aspects of best practice to encourage walking, cycling and other public transport use and act as showcases for other towns wishing to promote greater travel choice." Darlington, Peterborough and Worcester were selected from applications by 51 local authorities who submitted expressions of interest. They were selected on the basis of fully worked-up plans to deliver a sustainable transport scheme aiming to produce innovative school, work and personal travel plans; cycle lanes and improved cycle parking; better conditions for walking; and improved bus services.[310]

316. **It would not be appropriate for us to spell out the individual measures required to achieve the Government's ambitious cycling targets, although we were particularly impressed by the segregation of cyclists from road traffic we witnessed in Odense. If the Government were to achieve its target of trebling cycling in the period 2000–2010 (and there are very few signs that it will) that might achieve more in the fight against obesity than any individual measure we recommend within this report. So we would like the Department of Health to have a strategic input into transport policy and we believe it would be an important symbolic gesture of the move from a sickness to a health service if the Department of Health offered funding to support the Department for Transport's sustainable transport town pilots.**

317. As the submissions from Living Streets and SUSTRANS made clear, what is needed is a wholesale cultural change to a country where people are more active. Town planning needs to prioritise pedestrians and cyclists rather than road vehicles; a strip of white line at the side of a busy trunk road does not constitute a safe cycle route.

318. Sustrans, in partnership with the Children's Play Council and Transport 2000, has supported Home Zones schemes, where groups of streets are designed and laid out so that car users do not have priority over other users, with cars travelling at little more than walking pace. The design enables people to use the streets as a social space, meaning that children can play outside, neighbours can socialise and the local communities can take control of their own environments.[311]

319. There are other impediments to active travel in addition to the transport network and services. Services located in out-of-town sites where access is only easy by car promote a sedentary lifestyle and "help 'lock-in' car dependence."[312] The Social Exclusion Unit's report into transport and social exclusion indicated that from the mid 1970s to the late 1980s, total distance travelled for food shopping increased by 60%.[313] Whilst transport policies are necessary and important, the wider planning of communities also needs to change. There seem to be no regulations in place requiring active travel and recreation opportunities for all new housing developments; these are still being built with no consideration of the need for safe walking and cycling routes to school.

---

310 Department for Transport News Release 2003/0172

311 Ev 111

312 Ev 111

313 Ev 164 (Living Streets)

320. Many commentators argue that a national transport plan would be useful to promote and facilitate active methods of transport. Sustrans contended that obesity was a symptom of the way the physical environment had been planned and that therefore they would like to see changes that encouraged active forms of travel, such as higher parking charges and improved cycling routes. Sustrans, the National Heart Forum, the International Obesity Taskforce and others argued that a health impact assessment should be made on all transport project proposals and policies before implementation.

321. **There will be profound economic as well as health costs to be paid if the current obesity epidemic continues unchecked. Major planning proposals and transport projects are already subject to environmental impact assessment; we believe that it would be appropriate if a health impact assessment were also a statutory requirement. This would enable health to be integrated into the planning procedure and help bring about the sort of creative, joined-up solution which is required. This may seem a cumbersome and drastic step but we believe that only such strong measures will help reverse the dramatic decline in everyday activity that has occurred in recent decades.**

The workplace

322. Employers also have a role to play in encouraging activity. We were surprised not to receive a single memorandum from any industry not directly involved in obesity, or any umbrella organization representing the interests of industry, in the course of our inquiry. The problems of overweight and obesity are already having a substantial impact on business. For example, back pain is the largest single cause of days lost from work; obesity is a known contributor to back pain, as is a general lack of fitness.

323. Our predecessor Committee, in the course of its public health inquiry, visited Cuba, a country with remarkably good health outcomes given its relatively tiny health expenditure as compared with the UK.[314] One of the features of public health in Cuba is the extent to which workplaces encourage employees to take part in physical activity. It is true that there are isolated examples of similar practice within England, but they are the exception rather than the rule.

324. Sport England suggested that tax incentives could be provided to employers that provided gym membership to their staff.[315] We believe that this is an area that could be explored but we also recognise that there are many simple measures that could be taken to raise the energy output of employees at work. The NAO report *Tackling Obesity in England* noted the example of research by Glasgow University and Glasgow Health Board which aimed to test "whether incidental activity could be incorporated into the daily routines of members of the public." Simply by putting signs on the escalators encouraging stair use to maintain fitness, stair use increased by 15–17%.[316]

325. The settings for heating and air conditioning in offices affect the amount of energy the body uses. Commercial canteens, like schools, can provide healthy or unhealthy food; simply offering better information on, for example, the calorie content of different meals

---

314 Health Committee, Second Report of Session 2000-01, *Public Health*, HC 30, para 21

315 Appendix 19

316 *Tackling Obesity in England*, p 35

might offer a start. As we have already seen, employers can make cycling, walking or running easier for their employees by offering appropriate facilities.

326. Little seems to have been done to address the problems of sedentary behaviour in the workplace. Yet, as the working patterns of modern society have drastically altered, and as manual labour has dwindled, the office-bound workplace, with its desk, chair and computer terminal has become the norm for millions of people.

327. In the USA, one major company, Sprint Telecoms, has recently opened a 200 acre headquarters building designed to make its employees lose weight by forcing them to walk everywhere. The car parks have been built ten minutes walk away from the offices; staircases are airy and inviting; the lifts are slow and small. Sprint argues that reducing obesity will reduce absenteeism and improve the performance of its employees.[317]

328. **We recommend that the Department of Health, in conjunction with the Department for Work and Pensions and the Department of Trade and Industry first organises a major conference to promote awareness of obesity in the work-place and then engages in an ongoing process of consultation to see how measures can be taken to address sedentary behaviour. We recommend that these Departments consult with the Treasury to see what fiscal incentives can be provided to promote active travel.**

329. **We also recommend that the public sector looks to set an example in finding creative ways of encouraging activity in everyday life, and that this is built into a PSA target for each Department.**

Strategic direction

330. Some memoranda queried whether adequate structures existed to promote and implement measures to facilitate healthy lifestyles. Len Almond from the BHF National Centre for Physical Activity and Health called for a much-needed strategic platform to promote physical activity which would involve an alliance of interested organisations to plan the direction and lead on strategy.[318] He suggested: "at present there is no organisation that represents the interests of mass participation in health promoting physical activity in England. Consequently, there are no national strategic plans to promote physical activity for health."[319] It is clear however that in order to increase levels of physical activity, policies must make it easier for people to be more active as part of their daily routine—primarily through promoting active transport—and must encourage people to be more active in their recreation time.

331. Our predecessor Committee's report into *Public Health* recommended that the Government should appoint advisers to co-ordinate the work of all departments in delivering the sport and health agenda. The Government rejected this proposal but partly in response to our recommendation, and following findings in *Game Plan*, an Activity Co-ordination Team (ACT), was created and co-chaired by the Minister for Public Health and the Minister for Sport, with senior representatives from the following Departments:

317 "Architects join fight against the flab", BBC News website, 27 March 2003.
318 Ev 106
319 Ev 103

Health; Culture, Media and Sport; Education and Skills; Environment, Food and Rural Affairs; Work and Pensions; Office of the Deputy Prime Minister; Home Office; and Treasury. In addition, there were representatives from No. 10 Downing Street, Sport England, the Local Government Association, the New Opportunities Fund and the Health Development Agency. There was an interval of almost seven months between the recommendation in *Game Plan* that a board co-ordinating activity should be created, and the first meeting in July 2003 of the ACT. As we write this report it has met on five occasions.[320]

332. The practical steps it is hoped ACT will take will be to:

- Innovate, introducing change where there is supporting evidence and available funding—this should give early impetus to the work.

- Pull together evidence and present it—jointly with outside sporting and health organisations—as part of a positive communication strategy, disseminating evidence and best practice.

- Test and evaluate interventions where evidence is not strong, including external factors relating to increased participation, such as crime reduction—where the timescale might be longer.

- Identify sources of funding.

- Gather comprehensive data on participation and fitness regularly.[321]

333. The ACT, we were told, will produce "a three-year delivery plan by Spring 2004" which will seek to drive up mass participation. The ACT will present a progress report of its work later this year. In addition to this, the Department of Health is working to establish nine Local Exercise Pilots based in PCTs, whose aim will be to test different community approaches to increasing levels of and access to physical activity. The Department of Health pointed to a number of initiatives showing fruitful joint working between departments, such as the Healthy Schools initiative (joint Department of Health/Department for Education and Skills) and the Young People's Development Pilot Programme.

334. We welcome the creation of the Activity Co-ordination Team though we regret it took so long for it to begin its work. Anything that co-ordinates Government activity in this complex and challenging field is worthwhile. We await with interest the publication of its first report. We recommend that its reports explicitly link its activity to the Government's specific targets on activity both in schools and in the community.

---

320 HC Deb, 30 March 2004, col. 131 W

321 www.culture.gov.uk

The role of the NHS

Prevention of obesity

335. Prevention must clearly be the primary focus of any efforts to address the problem of obesity, as we have received compelling evidence suggesting that obesity, once established, is extremely hard to treat.[322] Much of the written evidence we received supported a policy focus centred on prevention, with the National Heart Forum arguing that "on the basis of current evidence and technologies there is very limited scope to reverse or 'cure' obesity in individuals."[323] We hope that the recommendations set out above will enable people to make healthy lifestyle choices, and that in turn these choices will allow trends in overweight and obesity to be stabilised in the short term, and reversed in the long term. However the health service clearly has an important role to play in backing up these environmental measures with explicit support for prevention.

336. PCTs, as well as commissioning health services for their local populations, have an explicit role in improving public health. To this end, we might have expected to receive evidence of a number of community-based initiatives geared to preventing obesity. However, we were struck in this inquiry, as in our inquiry into *Sexual Health*, by the fact that we received very little evidence on strategic prevention within the NHS. In fact, we received only one memorandum from a PCT public health lead, and none at all from Strategic Health Authorities, despite their responsibility for overseeing the delivery of public health services for the whole of their areas.

337. When we asked Department of Health officials how many PCTs currently had an obesity lead actively working on tackling the problem in their local area, they were not able to answer. **The Department agreed that Strategic Health Authorities (SHAs) should have information about local work on obesity at their fingertips, and we recommend that a survey of action on obesity, both at PCT and SHA level, should be undertaken as part of the ongoing work on the forthcoming White Paper on public health.**

338. A recent report by the independent health information organisation, Dr Foster, showed that strategic action on obesity seemed at best patchy:

> Although most Primary Care Organisations (PCOs)[324] had some form of publicly stated policy with regard to obesity, there was enormous variation between areas with some having highly developed policies, whilst in other areas the issue was given relatively little emphasis.

> Most PCO policy on tackling obesity is framed in the context of tackling CHD. The analysis of Local Development Plans showed that 30% of areas had well developed strategies in this area.

> In some areas, there was little more than a passing mention of obesity in Local Development Plans. For example, Harrow PCT has no detailed obesity strategy,

---

322 For example, see Appendix 33 (Dr Sheila McKenzie).

323 Ev 113

324 Including Primary Care Trusts, Local Health Boards in Wales and Scotland, and Health and Social Services Boards in Northern Ireland.

neither is obesity tackled specifically in its action plan for CHD … Cambridge City PCT also makes no reference to the prevention or treatment of obesity within other identified areas for action, e.g. CHD.[325]

339. Amanda Avery, a community dietician with Greater Derby PCT, told us that within PCTs there was not necessarily the flexibility needed to tackle the problem of obesity. She argued that:

> Drug budgets could be considerably reduced if obesity was better addressed. Unfortunately, it is quite difficult to transfer monies from a PCT's prescribing budget to help fund other initiatives to address obesity. All the emphasis is currently on guidance as to how to use drugs but not on guidance as to how to prevent their use in the first instance.[326]

340. Ms Avery also suggested that the structural changes in the NHS in recently years had led to difficulties around partnership working with other organisations:

> People who championed the obesity cause perhaps moved on. Within our PCT there are good examples of partnership working, but continuity is required over a number of years to establish good outcomes.[327]

341. The failure of PCTs fully to embrace the public health agenda seems also to be reflected more widely. Melanie Johnson told us of her view that there needed to be "fuller development of public health at the PCT level",[328] and the recent Wanless report also made several remarks in this area. It firstly highlighted the "disruptive impact" of the recent reorganisation of NHS structures on public health, arguing that the size of PCTs, and the capacity and dispersal of the public health workforce, had led in some areas to insufficient "critical mass" to fulfil public health responsibilities.[329] The creation of 303 PCTs from 95 Health Authorities has meant that public health resources within each PCT are now considerably smaller, and an increase in corporate responsibilities for each Director of Public Health has resulted in "a reduction in their ability to undertake and practise public health work."[330] Public health teams are now much smaller than they were previously, and with relatively high vacancy rates, many PCTs now 'share' their Directors of Public Health.

342. Derek Wanless reported "A survey commissioned by the Department of Health in 2002–03 to identify the capacity and development needs of PCT and Strategic Health Authorities found that the Specialist public health workforce was thinly distributed and unequally spread"[331], and some PCTs reported that the support provided for public health by SHAs was "variable"[332]. To counter these problems, he recommended that the Department should "reinforce the role of SHAs in relation to the performance

325 Dr Foster, *Obesity Management in the UK*, available at www.drfoster.co.uk.

326 Ev 351

327 Q 1101

328 Q1299

329 Derek Wanless, *Securing Good Health for the Whole Population*, Final Report, HM Treasury, February 2004

330 Ibid, p 45

331 Ibid, p 45

332 Ibid, p 49

management of the public health function within PCTs", and also that the Healthcare Commission "should develop a robust mechanism for the performance assessment of the public health role of PCTs and SHAs."[333]

343. **We feel strongly that Primary Care Trusts should be taking a more active role in preventing obesity, and urge the Government to ensure that PCTs have the capacity, competency and incentive to fulfil their crucial obligation to safeguard the public health of the local communities they serve. We also endorse the recommendation of the Wanless report that the Healthcare Commission should develop a robust mechanism for assessing performance of both PCTs and Strategic Health Authorities with respect to public health.**

Treatment of obesity

344. Dr Nick Finer, a consultant in obesity medicine at Addenbrooke's Hospital, Cambridge, stressed to us that "even the most successful prevention policies cannot address the current burden of ill health related to obesity, nor obviate the need now, or in the future, for appropriate medical care for the obese."[334] However, when we asked about the provision of such services, we were informed by the Department that the responsibility for ensuring provision of obesity services rested exclusively with PCTs. Worryingly, it was not only in strategic action to prevent obesity that PCTs, and the NHS more broadly, appeared to be failing. The evidence we received pointed repeatedly to the gross inadequacy of services currently available to tackle obesity within the NHS, as articulated by Dr Ian Campbell, a GP with a special interest in obesity:

> Whilst no-one would disagree that it is important to prevent obesity, particularly among children, I just find it inconceivable that we should reach a situation where we are not able to offer treatment to those who are already obese, which is about 10 million people.[335]

345. Sally Hayes, of North West Leeds PCT, described the current situation in even more stark terms, contending that "at present most of the NHS has no systematic approach for the management of obesity at any level of BMI."[336]

346. The problems appear to have originated with a lack of prioritisation within PCTs, and to have filtered through every level of service provision. TOAST argued that the vast majority of PCT teams were unaware of their obese patients and "frankly uninterested and unaware of the aetiology of the problem."[337] This view was supported by Roche, who maintained that there was "little motivation within PCTs to ensure that weight management is offered to patients" since obesity is seen as a "lifestyle" not a medical issue.[338] The Dr Foster research showed that over half of primary care organisations in the UK did not have organised weight-management clinics within their local areas, and even in

---

333   Ibid, p 50

334   Ev 329

335   Q1046

336   Ev 354

337   Ev 372

338   Appendix 6

those areas that did, such clinics were available on average through only a quarter of GP practices. According to Roche, "obesity does not rank very highly as an area of interest to GPs", a view which was re-emphasised by Sally Hayes:

> At present, primary care professionals are offering short term support to people who are obese within current resources which may include diet, activity and behavioural strategies. Unfortunately this is often on an ad hoc basis with little structure to these key interactions.[339]

347. Obesity is a complex medical problem, and it is clear that superficial interventions, such as the distribution of a diet sheet to an obese patient, are unlikely to work. Specialist skills and knowledge are needed fully to engage with obesity as a psychological and behavioural as well as a physiological problem. It has been likened by some to alcoholism, and requires similarly holistic treatment programmes.

348. Professor John Baxter, a consultant bariatric surgeon, described his constant amazement at the fact that other doctors referring patients to him for bariatric surgery appeared to know so little about obesity, and evidence from those actually working in primary care supported this view. Louise Mann, a practice nurse at the Gable House Surgery in Wiltshire, told us that "as nurses, we do not get any training at all in weight management in our training. In primary care and with our practice, we did weight management, but very much in an *ad hoc* way, with no instruction at all."[340]

349. This is perhaps particularly concerning given that many of our witnesses were in agreement that primary care was the best level at which to tackle obesity. The National Obesity Forum argued that the "vast majority of overweight and obese people are encountered within primary care, either seeking help directly for their weight problem, or indirectly because of a related medical condition", and maintained that primary care was the best place to offer intervention and concentrate funds and efforts.[341] And according to Colin Waine, Visiting Professor of Primary Care at the University of Sunderland, "about 75% of the population see their general practitioner in one year and approximately 90% over a five-year period. Thus the opportunities exist to identify opportunistically people at high risk and likely to benefit" from treatment. Dr Waine went on to argue that this was in fact one of the great strengths of the British system of primary care.[342] Research commissioned by Roche suggested that patients were reluctant to discuss their weight pro-actively, and would prefer their health care professional to raise the issue. However, further research found that general practitioners were unlikely to raise the issue of obesity during a health consultation.[343]

350. The Counterweight project, a pilot obesity management study being trialled in 80 general practices, is attempting to evaluate the usefulness of setting up specialised obesity-management clinics within a general practice setting, following specialised training and using tailored protocols. The clinicians, who do not necessarily need to be GPs, follow

---

339 Ev 354

340 Q1082

341 Ev 318

342 Q1063

343 Appendices 6 and 7

protocols setting out different evidence-based 'lifestyle approaches' to obesity management. The programme will be fully audited in each practice after two years, and will measure changes in clinician knowledge, attitudes, perceived confidence and willingness to treat obesity, as well as changes in practice approaches to obesity management and weight-screening rates. The primary end point for the patient intervention programme will be the percentage of patients achieving $\geq$5% and $\geq$ 10 % weight loss. While the final conclusions of the programme will not be known for some time, the preliminary results from the intervention programme indicate that clinically beneficial weight loss can be achieved in high-risk obese patients in the primary care setting.[344]

351. However, service providers maintained that resources to provide structured, long-term interventions to tackle obesity in primary care were simply not available. Dr Campbell felt that GPs would be "up in arms" if they were instructed to institute routine measurement of BMI, and stated categorically that there was no point in measuring BMI without sufficient resources to address obesity where it is identified:

> To try to put this into context, my own practice is 4,500 patients, and we have identified 483 who are clinically obese. I could not start to treat all of those tomorrow, so just measuring it is one thing. You need therefore the resources to do something about it.[345]

352. The Counterweight Project told us that it deliberately did not give practices extra funding, relying, in the words of a practice nurse, "on the good will of GPs".[346] We also heard how a 15-month project to develop a service for weight management within four GP practices in the Leeds North West area also risked being abandoned as it could not secure ongoing funding.[347]

353. In contradiction of the Public Health Minister's argument that the new GP contract provided sufficient incentives for health promotion, Dr Campbell told us that out of a possible 1,000 quality points GPs could gain, only three could be acquired by measuring body mass index.[348] None related purely to the treatment of obesity. Dr Campbell characterised this failure of the new GP contract to incentivise GPs to treat obesity as a significant mistake.

354. Our witnesses argued compellingly that improving obesity services within primary care was not an aspiration that was entirely out of reach. Dr Campbell suggested that programmes to train primary care clinicians in obesity management, like the Counterweight project and that being undertaken by Leeds North West PCT, would not need to be extended to all primary care practices, but that targeted training need only be offered to interested GPs. Trained GPs with a specialist interest in obesity could then provide specialist obesity services within their own practices, and other practices could also refer to them, as an intermediary between primary and secondary care.

344 Ev 344-46
345 Q1064
346 Q1077
347 Q1084
348 Q1066

355. We feel that this country's well developed network of primary care providers, local GPs, provides a unique resource for health promotion and for the identification and management of patients who are overweight or obese. However, managing weight problems sensitively and successfully requires specialist skills, and we are concerned by suggestions that obesity is viewed by many clinicians as a lifestyle issue rather than a serious health problem requiring active management to prevent dire health consequences. We deplore the low priority given to obesity by the new GP contract. We hope that NICE guidance on the prevention, identification, evaluation, treatment and weight maintenance of overweight and obesity, currently expected in Summer 2006, will go some way towards increasing the priority of obesity within general practice, as well as helping primary care practitioners develop and improve the services they provide in this difficult area. The Government should also ensure that within each PCT area there is at least one specialist primary care obesity clinic, probably supported by a range of different health professionals, to which GPs can refer any patients they identify as needing specialist support to address a developing or existing weight problem.

356. Weight management within primary care may not necessarily need to take place in traditional primary care settings such as the GP surgery, or even be carried out by GPs. The majority of practices in the Counterweight project, for example, ran nurse-led clinics under the supervision of a GP. Community dieticians can also play an important part, and organisations representing community pharmacists have submitted evidence stating that they are keen to play an increased role in dealing with obesity; and that they have developed thinking in this area, building on an existing scheme for diabetes testing.[349] In Finland we noted moves to make testing for diabetes available in a much wider range of settings. **We recommend that, in establishing primary care obesity clinics, PCTs should fully explore the possibilities of using less traditional models of service delivery, involving clinicians from across the professional spectrum, from nurses to pharmacists to dieticians. The full range of interventions available to treat obesity includes diet, lifestyle, medical treatment and surgical treatment.**

357. **We also took some interesting evidence from commercial slimming organisations. We recommend that the NHS examines whether their expertise can be brought to bear in devising strategies to combat obesity holistically.**

358. Although primary care provides the best starting point for treating people with weight problems, more specialist care is clearly necessary for some patients, particularly those with severe and complex problems relating to their obesity, including, amongst others, patients with metabolic and cardiovascular disease whose treatment will need to involve an holistic approach to their medical needs; those suffering from sleep apnoea syndrome; those requiring peri-operative care where weight loss may be needed to minimise risk and optimise outcome; and those with life-threatening morbid obesity.

359. The evidence we received universally pointed to a dire lack of specialist obesity care provision in the NHS. Sally Hayes, of North West Leeds PCT, stated that currently "the secondary care service for morbid obesity has a closed waiting list."[350] Dr Nick Finer, a

349 Appendix 26 (The Pharmaceutical Services Negotiating Committee); Appendix 31 (Lloydspharmacy)

350 Ev 354

consultant obesity physician, argued that "secondary care cannot effectively contribute to the management of obesity since it hardly exists."[351] Interestingly, we heard that there have in fact recently been specific directives aimed at the treatment of obesity in secondary and tertiary care. Services for morbid obesity were defined in the Specialised Services National Definitions Set (2nd Edition) No. 35, released by the Department in December 2002. These identified specialised treatment activity that should be subject to collaborative commissioning arrangements including: "an integral management approach … aimed at weight loss and weight maintenance … drawn up by a multi-disciplinary team to meet the needs and requirements of each individual patient." However, Dr Finer argued that in his own area of Anglia, as well as elsewhere in the UK, "these services remain unimplemented, with no process or individual responsible for their implementation as yet operational."[352]

360. Dr Finer reported that the existence of both of the clinics he ran had always been dependent upon research funding, and that both clinics struggled "to receive explicit funding from Primary Care Trusts."[353] He also described the significant mismatch between demand and capacity. At his Luton clinic, he could see about 250 new patients a year. At Addenbrooke's the capacity was only 80 new patients a year. However, the clinics regularly received five times as many referrals as this, and even this figure did not take account of a vast amount of untapped demand. Dr Finer estimated that the current prevalence of obesity meant that within the catchment area of a typical hospital serving a population of 300,000, about 130,000 adults would be overweight or obese, 53,000 obese (BMI>30), and about 3,500 morbidly obese (BMI>40). This means that even if specialist obesity treatment were only to be offered to all patients with morbid obesity, Dr Finer's clinic would require a 14-fold increase in capacity.[354]

361. Oversubscription to the clinic recently forced Dr Finer to run 'group' consultations, which were not well received by patients, and also, more worryingly, to close his clinics to new patients when waiting lists got too long:

> The problem has always been how to meet the demand which is there, with the lack of resources. At Luton … over the last seven or eight years the only way of managing referrals was to shut the clinic to referrals. I have been at Addenbrooke's now full-time for a year, and I run a clinic that is primarily resourced from my appointment as a university appointment. Without my doing a large number of extra clinics to see these new patients, I would have lost Addenbrooke's Hospital its third star probably six months ago.[355]

362. The Department told us that there were only ten obesity clinics in England, and that these were not evenly distributed.[356] According to Dr Finer, all of these clinics had waiting lists of "at least 12 months".[357] To put this in context it is worth noting that the

351 Ev 329
352 Ev 329
353 Ev 328
354 Ev 329
355 Q1047
356 Q60
357 Q1051

Government aims to achieve a maximum wait of three months for an outpatient appointment in any specialty by 2005, and interim targets for March 2004 were set at no more than four months for an outpatient appointment.[358] However, when discussing with us the number and availability of specialist obesity clinics, Department of Health officials did not seem concerned about the low numbers, and stated that "whether there should be more is a decision that needs to be taken through PCTs in consultation with other local commissioners as to the need."[359]

363. **Obesity is a serious medical problem. Although in common with other illnesses, its prevention and some first-line management can be delivered within a primary care setting, patients with more entrenched or complex problems need prompt access to specialist medical care. Childhood obesity is a worrying and increasingly common subset of this illness, and children in particular need specialist care. Yet specialist obesity services seem to be an almost entirely neglected area of the NHS, apparently exempt from Government initiatives to push down waiting times despite their obvious importance in preventing a large range of other debilitating and costly diseases. We therefore recommend that the Government provides funding for the large scale expansion of obesity services in secondary care, underpinned by careful management to ensure that the service provision is matched to need. The Government's maximum waiting time targets must apply to all of these services.**

364. The treatment of children with obesity is, if anything, more important than that for adults, as habits set down in childhood are likely to form the pattern for the rest of a person's life. However, Dr Finer told us that specialist services for obese children were "even patchier" than the virtually non-existent provision for adults, a view endorsed by Dr Mary Rudolf, a consultant paediatrician with a specialist interest in obesity:

> There is a dire lack of services within the NHS for the management of childhood obesity. Our experience in Leeds is likely to be typical of the rest of the country. There is no specialist service even for the grossly obese. A minority of these children are seen in the Regional Endocrinology Service (and only if they are likely to have medical problems resulting from their obesity). They are seen briefly and only very periodically for a "medical check" but no real intervention. The hospital paediatric dietetic department is so limited that there is a ruling that no child may receive dietetic advice about their obesity even if they are on medication for the problem.[360]

365. In June 2003 the waiting list for the specialist obesity service for children at Bart's and the London Trust stood at 11 months and rising.[361]

366. **We were appalled to learn of the desperate inadequacy of treatment and support services for obese children. Steps must be taken to ensure that obese children and young people have prompt access to specialist treatment wherever they live.**

---

358 *Improvement, Expansion and Reform – the next three years – Priorities and Planning Framework 2003-2006,* Department of Health

359 Q60

360 Ev 329; Appendix 4

361 Appendix 33

367. Recent research carried out by the Peninsula Medical School has suggested that overweight and obesity are now becoming so commonplace amongst children that even parents are failing to notice when their own children become overweight or obese. In a survey of 300 British families, only 25% of parents with overweight children recognised that their children were overweight. No fathers identified their sons as overweight, even when they were, and, perhaps even more disturbingly, 33% of mothers and 57% of fathers described their children as 'normal' when in fact they were obese.[362] As treatment is only possible once a problem has been identified, this represents a worrying trend. We were also told by Professor Jane Wardle, of the Health Behaviour Unit at University College London, that parental concern about children developing eating problems may be overly biased towards eating disorders such as anorexia and bulimia:

> I think parents feel exceptionally responsible if their children develop eating disorders. I think probably they feel slightly less responsible if their children develop obesity, even though that may not be the justifiable allocation of responsibility.[363]

368. We feel that the school nursing system offers a valuable opportunity to correct this through a programme of routine measurement of BMI throughout a child's school career. The Children's Minister, Margaret Hodge, expressed reservations about the possibility that such a measure could stigmatise overweight and obese children. We are confident that this could be overcome, through the adoption of a sensitive approach whereby rather than singling out individuals, all school children are weighed and measured once a year, and their BMI results sent in confidence to their parents together with, if appropriate, advice on how to modify diet and exercise patterns. Not only would this system identify children who are already overweight or obese, but it could target those at the top end of the 'normal' range of BMI to prevent further weight gain. As the Public Health Minister reassured us that every school now had access to a school nurse, we are confident that such a scheme could be administered within existing resources.

369. **We recommend that throughout their time at school, children should have their Body Mass Index measured annually at school, perhaps by the school nurse, a health visitor, or other appropriate health professional. The results should be sent home in confidence to their parents, together with, where appropriate, advice on lifestyle, follow-up, and referral to more specialised services. Where appropriate, BMI measurement could be carried out alongside other health care interventions which are delivered at school, for example inoculation programmes. Care will need to be taken to avoid stigmatising children who are overweight or obese, but given that research indicates that many parents are no longer even able to identify whether their children are overweight or not, this seems to us a vital step in tackling obesity.**

370. The National Institute for Clinical Excellence (NICE) has published guidance supporting the use of the obesity drugs orlistat and sibutramine in certain, limited circumstances.[364] These drugs in no way represent a 'cure' for obesity, their success rate averaging a maximum of 5kg of weight loss per year of treatment, weight loss which is

---

362 *The Observer*, 14 March 2004

363 Q205

364 Nice Guidance No 22, Orlistat for the treatment of obesity in adults, 9 March 2001. Nice Guidance No 31, Sibutramine for the treatment of obesity in adults, 26 October 2001.

usually regained once treatment has stopped. For this reason, the conditions attached by NICE to use of these treatments stipulate that they must be supported by dietary and lifestyle changes. According to the Department's memorandum, estimated costs since the two products became available on the NHS are now approximately £31 million.[365]

371. Research carried out by Dr Foster concluded that 96% of PCTs were prepared to provide funding for drugs for the treatment of obesity, although 4% were not, despite the NICE guidelines. However, this does not necessarily provide a true picture of whether all patients who could potentially benefit from drug treatment are obtaining it, as this will depend on whether GPs are knowledgeable and confident enough to prescribe it, or whether patients are able to secure a referral to vastly over-subscribed specialist obesity clinics. Equally, although PCTs may have an official policy of funding the drugs, GPs may come under pressure to curtail their prescribing of obesity drugs to stay within cost limits, a situation described to us by Dr Campbell:

> Two days ago I received a letter from my own primary care trust saying that as a PCT we were quite high in our use of weight-loss medication, and we were to reconsider our practice policies. I cannot recall, in 15 years in general practice, receiving a letter questioning our prescribing of heart disease medication or diabetic medication; and this really typifies the prevailing attitude at the moment.[366]

372. We were dismayed to hear that a specialist GP who devoted much of his time to trying to tackle obesity in his local population was being put under pressure from his local PCT to reduce his prescribing of drugs to tackle obesity, despite these drugs having received approval from NICE, with the corresponding obligation on PCTs to provide funding for them. We were told by the same doctor that in 15 years of practice he had never received communications questioning his prescribing rates for drugs to treat heart disease or diabetes, two illnesses frequently caused by obesity. This provides a telling exposé of current attitudes towards obesity, whereby it is regarded by NHS decision-makers as a lifestyle problem for which treatment is an optional extra. We recommend that the Government takes urgent steps to tackle this subtle deprioritisation of obesity wherever it occurs in the NHS.

373. A more drastic option for treating obesity is through surgery. Obesity surgery, also described as bariatric surgery, can be either 'malabsorptive' or 'restrictive'. Malabsorptive surgery works by shortening the length of the digestive tract (gut) so that the amount of food absorbed by the body is reduced. This type of surgery involves creating a bypass by joining one part of the intestine to another. Restrictive surgery limits the size of the stomach so the person feels full after eating a small amount of food. This type of surgery can involve 'stapling' parts of the stomach together or fitting a tight band to make a small pouch for food to enter.[367] Currently, four types of obesity surgery are available: vertical banded gastroplasty, the Lap-Band system, Roux-en Y gastric bypass, or biliopancreatic diversion with a duodenal switch.

---

365 Ev 2

366 Q1036

367 Nice Technology Appraisal Guidance – No 46, Obesity Surgery, p 3, 19, July 2002

374. NICE have also given their approval for obesity surgery to be funded for NHS patients. Having reviewed 19 clinical trials and other evidence, NICE concluded that:

> surgery for people with morbid obesity is associated with significant weight loss that is maintained for at least 8 years, whereas there is little sustained weight loss with conventional treatment in this group of patients. Surgery is also associated with improved quality of life and reduced co-morbidities. There are significant risks attached to surgery, although these are thought to be outweighed by the benefits.[368]

However, Professor John Baxter, a consultant bariatric surgeon, told us that despite this recommendation obesity surgery services in the UK were 'third world' when compared with other developed countries. NICE's guidance suggested that the NHS should aim to build bariatric services up over the next eight years to around 4,000 procedures per year, from the 200–300 procedures performed in the UK at present. Professor Baxter felt this target number to be "manifestly too low".[369]

375. Based on the assumption that in the UK around 0.8% of males and 2% of females are morbidly obese, Professor Baxter argued that there were currently around 228,000 men and 570,000 women potentially suitable for surgery. If this were expanded to include all patients who had a BMI between 35 and 40 who had a co-morbid condition, this would push the target population up to 1.2 million. On top of this, Professor Baxter estimated that a further 5,000–8,000 patients would become morbidly obese each year. Even if only 5% of suitable patients opted for surgery, in his view a very conservative estimate, this would mean a current "backlog" of around 60,000 patients needing surgery immediately. Professor Baxter told us that the Swedish health service worked on the assumption that to maintain a "steady state", 500–1,000 procedures are needed per year per 500,000 population. Extrapolating this using UK data, around 25,000 procedures would be needed per year in this country, over six times the number recommended by NICE.[370]

376. Dr Finer supported Professor Baxter's view about the problems with obesity surgery:

> Obesity surgery remains virtually unfunded and unavailable to most eligible patients through the failure of district Health Authorities and now Primary Care Trusts to implement NICE guidance.[371]

377. Professor Baxter described provision of bariatric surgery as a "postcode service" and warned that Strategic Health Authorities were now "starting to panic about how to provide this service."[372] He told us that waiting lists were very long in all centres. For his service, in Swansea, the waiting list was one year for an outpatients appointment, followed by three years' wait for surgery, giving a total wait of four years. Another impediment to access was that many suitable patients were not being referred simply because their GPs were ignorant about bariatric surgery. The huge mismatch between capacity and need was shown by

---

368 Ibid

369 Ev 332

370 Ibid

371 Ev 329

372 Q1058

Professor Baxter's estimate that at least 300 obesity surgeons were needed, compared with the 13 or 14 currently practising.

378. In the United States, we met with two bariatric surgeons who explained that bariatric surgery was a rapidly increasing speciality there. Last year there were 103,000 bariatric operations performed in the US and this figure is projected to rise to 126,000 this year. While up until two years ago, these operations were only carried out in large specialist university hospitals, now almost every private hospital, both large and small, performs the operations.

379. **Bariatric surgery is in no way a panacea for the current obesity epidemic. Rather it is a high-risk, invasive surgical procedure that represents a last line of defence for people with life-threatening morbid obesity. However as the number of people suffering from morbid obesity in England looks set to increase, it is an option that needs to be made available to all those who need it, and it is unacceptable that in some parts of the UK patients with a life-threatening condition are having to wait as long as four years for bariatric surgery. We hope that the measures we have recommended to improve provision of specialist obesity services in both primary and secondary care will help to address the problem that many patients are not referred for bariatric surgery simply because their local doctors are not aware that it is an option. However, the NHS needs also to ensure that adequate service capacity is in place fully to meet need, which is patently not the case at present. The Government must devote protected resources to ensuring that bariatric surgery is available to all those who need it, and should issue guidelines for the strategic development of services across the country, to eliminate the current postcode provision of obesity surgery.**

380. As well as medical and surgical approaches, it is vital that the psychological and behavioural aspects of obesity are addressed. As TOAST pointed out in their written evidence, there are a multitude of reasons why people may overeat, many of them linked to underlying psychological factors:

We have asked a variety of groups why they think obese people overeat. The following list is typical of the answers given:

Boredom	Guilt
Anger	Shame
Stress	Because it's there
Loneliness	Pressure from other people
Happiness	Going to start a diet tomorrow
Revenge	Frustration
Depression	It's Sunday
Addiction	Pleasure
Habit	Unloved
Not appreciated	Unfulfilled
Tired	Unsatisfied
Unhappy	To celebrate
Comfort	Holidays[373]

381. TOAST argued that amongst some groups, obesity was comparable to addictive habits such as smoking or alcohol dependence:

> For many types of obese [people] there is a strong link to the problems of those with a drink problem; many talk of sometimes feeling out of control around food … All the alcohol treatment programmes we know of use some form of counselling within their treatment profile. They recognise that the alcohol is often used as a coping mechanism, to drown sorrows, for swallowing anger, blotting out the pain, to be part of the crowd. Many overeaters will recognise these behaviours and reasons for over consuming. Alcohol treatment programmes help people to recognise why they have been over consuming and to find other coping mechanisms, helping clients build belief in them.[374]

382. TOAST and the Royal College of Psychiatrists both argued strongly that multidisciplinary teams to treat obesity must involve a range of professionals properly equipped to address the psychological and behavioural aspects of obesity, including counsellors, psychiatrists, psychotherapists, psychologists and family therapists.[375] **We feel it is vital that advances in medical and surgical treatment of obesity should be supported by equivalent development of services to address the psychological and**

---

373 Ev 372

374 Ev 372

375 Appendix 40

behavioural aspects of obesity. All those receiving treatment for obesity, whether in a primary or in secondary care setting, should have access to psychological support provided by an appropriate professional, whether this is a psychiatrist, psychologist, psychotherapist, counsellor, or family therapist.

Prioritisation within the NHS

383. While we agree that the obesity epidemic has, in contrast to other public health concerns which may come to prominence very rapidly, manifested itself gradually and insidiously over a number of years, we were a little surprised to hear the Public Health Minister, Melanie Johnson, argue that it had "caught us all slightly unawares."[376] While it is clear that the Government and the NHS are at present unprepared to deal with this problem on the scale at which it now presents itself, obesity has been recognised as a serious threat to the nation's public health by experts and governments alike for several decades. In 1976, nearly 30 years ago, a report by a joint Department of Health and Social Security and Medical Research Council group highlighted the problem in unequivocal terms:

> We are unanimous in our belief that obesity is a hazard to health and a detriment to well being. It is common enough to constitute one of the most important medical and public health problems of our time, whether we judge importance by shorter expectation of life, increased morbidity, or cost to the community in terms of both money and anxiety.[377]

384. Twelve years ago, the 1992 White Paper *The Health of the Nation* identified targets for obesity reduction. These targets were not met, and obesity increased rather than decreased during this period. However, there were no obesity targets in the 1999 public health White Paper *Saving Lives*, an omission regarded by TOAST as deplorable: "With the obesity epidemic raging, obesity had been dropped, with no strategy being pursued to reduce or limit it."[378] When questioned about why this had happened, Department of Health officials responded that the issue of targets was a question for Ministers. In its memorandum, the Department argued that service-based targets within existing NSFs were sufficient:

> The Priorities and Planning Framework for 2003–06 includes targets for reducing CHD. One of these targets requires practice-based registers and systematic treatment regimes, including appropriate advice on diet, physical activity and smoking. This also covers the majority of patients at high risk of CHD, particularly those with hypertension, diabetes and a BMI greater than 30. In order to tackle health inequalities, the Priorities and Planning Framework also sets a target to contribute to a national reduction in death rates from CHD focusing on the 20% of areas with the highest rates of CHD, and this should encourage action on obesity in disadvantaged areas. The Priorities and Planning Framework has also set a target to increase breastfeeding initiation rates by 2 percentage points each year, particularly among disadvantaged groups.

---

376 Q1301

377 Cited in Appendix 18 (Royal College of General Practitioners)

378 Ev 369

Standard One of the NSF for CHD relates to the reduction of coronary risk factors in the population and requires that all NHS bodies will have agreed and be contributing to the delivery of a local programme of effective policies on promoting healthy eating, increasing physical activity and reducing overweight and obesity and have quantified data on the programme by April 2002.[379]

385. Speaking to the *Health Service Journal*, Melanie Johnson, the Public Health Minister, expressed her view that the current package of measures to tackle obesity,—which she listed as the school fruit scheme, the Five-a-day fruit and vegetable initiative, and the as yet unpublished Food and Health Action Plan—when taken together "amounted to a strategy" to tackle obesity.[380]

386. However, none of these things has any direct connection to NHS services to prevent and treat obesity. And although the Government has often cited a reluctance within the health service for more targets and central directives, we in fact received a substantial body of evidence from those working within the NHS who argued strongly in support of a national service framework specifically addressing obesity. Significantly, this call has come both from clinicians and from those involved in NHS management. Dr Ian Campbell, a GP, told us that:

> The impact of a national service framework should not be underestimated within the world of general practice. The National Institute for Clinical Excellence has made many pronouncements on weight management and the use of drugs for surgery, but they are only accepted at a distance by health authorities and not always acted upon; whereas national service frameworks are accepted as being directives that must be done, by which primary care services are judged; so it would have a huge impact on the service that followed.[381]

387. Sally Hayes, the CHD Lead at Leeds North West PCT supported this view, stating that an NSF in obesity "would help greatly" as "the setting of standards and targets does wake us up, as organisations".[382] She described her current means of securing one-off funding for obesity as "a mad scramble to try and bid for this and that", and told us that funding uncertainties prevented her project from being developed further, leading to de-motivation amongst staff involved in tackling obesity.[383]

388. According to the Institute of Human Nutrition at the University of Southampton, a key problem with the UK health system in relation to obesity was that there was "a notable absence of well-structured and validated care pathways" and that furthermore, "there is no formal budgetary responsibility at any level of care—community, primary, secondary or tertiary—for the identification of the overweight and the support and management of those identified as being at special risk."[384]

---

379 Ev 15-16

380 *Health Service Journal*, 6 November 2003, pp 26-27

381 Q1041

382 Q1075

383 Q1084

384 Appendix 32

389. Although the Department argued that the references to obesity within the NSFs for CHD and diabetes were sufficient to address obesity, we were told by the Counterweight Project that, ironically, those NSFs were in fact drawing resources *away* from the prevention and treatment of obesity, despite the indisputable link between obesity and both CHD and diabetes:

> The main barriers to continued provision of a structured approach to obesity management have been competing priorities and a lack of dedicated nurse time. Many practices however claim to be prioritising nurse and GP time to meet the national service frameworks for conditions such as diabetes and coronary heart disease. Ironically, many of these competing disease areas can be directly improved by obesity management.[385]

390. Dr Nick Finer, a consultant obesity physician, argued that the references to obesity within two NSFs were scant and ineffectual:

> Although there are odd little lines in the existing NSF to cardiology and diabetes, the fact that they are right down in the sub-sub-sections, means that to all intents and purposes they are ignored.[386]

391. Sally Hayes supported this view:

> Obesity is not specified enough within those standards and milestones. There are other things based on medication, on lifestyle. It is not specific enough really, and the targets are not specific enough.[387]

392. Dr Ian Campbell, in his capacity as Chairman of the National Obesity Forum, was one of many to recommend the appointment of a 'Fat Czar' to develop a central government strategy to tackle obesity on all fronts, in addition to the development of an Obesity National Service Framework and obesity targets for the NHS.

393. **The evidence we received during the course of this inquiry has convinced us that despite its overwhelming importance, obesity remains a low priority for the majority of service commissioners and providers in the NHS. The National Health Service has a responsibility both to take strategic action to prevent obesity, as part of its public health remit, and to provide adequate treatment for those already suffering from overweight or obesity, as it would for those suffering from any other medical condition. It appears to us to be failing in both of these areas, and this needs to change as a matter of urgency.**

394. **We are fully aware that obesity is mentioned in existing NSFs, but we believe that these scant mentions are woefully inadequate to provide a strategic framework through which to tackle what has been described as 'the biggest public health threat of the twenty-first century'. We also understand that a public health White Paper will be published in the summer, but again we fear that the extent and seriousness of the**

---

385 Ev 346

386 Q1040

387 Q1075

obesity problem will be lost by including obesity only as part of a wider umbrella of general public health initiatives.

395. We note the Government's reservations about committing to further National Service Frameworks, which they voiced in response to our report on *Sexual Health*. However, the current structure of the National Service Framework programme places too great an emphasis on tackling discrete disease areas, focusing on downstream consequences at the expense of the upstream contributors to these diseases, including obesity. Indeed, we heard compelling evidence that many general practices are unable to devote time to tackling obesity because of their obligation to meet targets in the Coronary Heart Disease and Diabetes NSFs, even though, ironically, many of these 'competing' disease areas can be directly improved by tackling obesity. And while it is clear that general public health problems, such as smoking, can be addressed within disease-based NSFs, the lack of obesity targets has led to this area being systematically neglected.

396. It is essential that, as part of the Government's wider strategy to tackle obesity, a dedicated framework document is produced to emphasise to a largely sceptical NHS the full scale and seriousness of this problem. The complexity of the challenge facing the NHS in this area, including the need to develop services and care pathways across all tiers of service delivery in a rapidly changing area of medicine, as well as to take the lead on prevention and health promotion, makes a detailed strategic framework vital. This document should build on existing work in this area, drawing together and emphasising the obesity measures already set out in the National Service Frameworks, and linking in with the ongoing work of NICE. Crucially, it must re-introduce realistic but stretching targets for reducing the prevalence of obesity and overweight over the next ten years, underpinned by more detailed, service-based targets, in particular bringing waiting times for specialist medical and surgical obesity services in line with all other NHS specialties. PCTs should be stringently performance-managed on their delivery of these targets.

4 Conclusion

397. Often the purpose of a select committee inquiry goes beyond the simple 'tick box' approach of making recommendations to Government and seeing how many are accepted. We believe that the very fact of our holding this inquiry has contributed (alongside many other important reports and studies) to the huge publicity that the subject of obesity has prompted over the last year or two, and has helped to raise its profile. *The Daily Telegraph* offered 177 articles on obesity in the year leading up to our inquiry and 337 in the year of our inquiry.

398. One of our witnesses argued that it might be helpful if more stigma attached to obesity so that people made more effort to lose excess weight.[388] We totally disagree with this suggestion. Nevertheless, we have observed an odd tension in society. The world of popular culture, teenage magazines, film, music and sport is usually dominated by fit and slim people. It is generally accepted that these are role models and that people aspire to emulate them. Yet the average person is remorselessly getting heavier and moving further and further away from the ideal. It is as if the pressure to conform to the stereotype, and failing, is pushing people in the opposite direction.

399. We have posited a wide range of measures in our report which attempt to address the issue of obesity. As many witnesses who appeared before us acknowledged, no single measure is likely to reverse the tide of obesity; a wide range of different measures is more likely to have an impact.

400. The rapid rise in obesity is now leading to a proliferation of meetings, conferences and pronouncements on this subject. This is in part extremely welcome in that it raises the awareness of the public, health professionals and policy makers in respect of a vitally important subject. However there is a danger that this could lead to policy overload, as different emphases are given—now on exercise, now on diet. There is a danger that this issue is characterised only within a polemical debate, stressing only the role of a 'devious food industry' on the one hand or the evils of the motor car or gameboy on the other. The evidence we heard suggests both 'energy in' and 'energy out' must be addressed, and indeed, part of the policy confusion is that there is inadequate liaison of policy response between the two 'sectors' of the obesity business. This can easily be exploited by vested interests resistant to change.

401. Many of the measures we recommend relating to physical activity would take years to implement, notably our call for a fundamental cultural change in urban planning to facilitate active travel and active workplaces. It would take even longer to measure the impact of these measures. Nevertheless, we believe it is vital that Government takes seriously its responsibilities to help people become more active.

402. We have commended the commitment and funding now being devoted to organised sport and physical activity in schools. Many of our other proposals would involve

---

388 Q195 (Professor Julian Peto)

substantial public expenditure, but the dire threat to public finances as well as public health if the obesity epidemic progresses unchecked persuades us that this expenditure is justifiable.

403. It would be very difficult to disaggregate the possible impact of any of the recommendations we make. We have argued for a coherent package of measures, addressing both sides of the energy equation. We believe they would have more chance of being effective if implemented in full rather than in a piecemeal fashion. However, it is clearly important that some steps are taken to monitor the effectiveness, and the cost-effectiveness of what we propose, in line with the recommendations of the Wanless report on public health. The National Audit Office undertook an influential and ground-breaking report on obesity in 2001. We know that they have maintained an interest in the subject thereafter. So we would like the National Audit Office to conduct further work on the value for money implications of measures taken to combat obesity, since this will be one of the greatest pressures on NHS resources over the coming decades. In calling for this, we also note the point made in the Scrutiny Unit analysis annexed to our report that there is a "severe lack" of official estimates of the costs of diseases relating to obesity. We recommend that the Department undertakes urgent work to establish better estimates of the cost of treating diseases to allow it to manage its resources more effectively.

404. We believe it is important to offer some perspective on the likely effectiveness of some of the short-term measures we propose in relation to food. One tool for doing this is provided by a substantial piece of research conducted by the investment bank J P Morgan. In a report published in April 2003, the bank investigated the possible impact of the growth of obesity on the food industry.[389] They looked from the perspective of the investor at the possible risks to the volumes of the food industry of greater regulation. Their findings are summarised in the table below:

389 J P Morgan, European Equity Research, *Food Manufacturing: The Big Issue*, pp. 15-21

Table 7: J P Morgan analysis of the impact of regulation on the food industry

Possible action	Likely impact on the food industry
Total ban on advertising of food and beverages to children on TV	"We think volumes would suffer. This is because not only are children significant consumers of the segment themselves, through 'pester power' they also drive broader retailing of the category … manufacturers would be faced with the double challenge of shifting the portfolio to healthier products while also finding alternative and innovative ways of selling these to children."
Labels having to have better nutritional information	"The US experience proves that labels containing more information about nutrition do not necessarily encourage people to adopt lower-calorie diets or reduce consumption." "We feel that nutritional labels on European food products may not change consumption patterns."
Targeting of super-size products	"These products carry a higher margin than regular products … were these products to become the target of regulators we believe it would have negative implications for volume growth."
Provision of warning labels for high-energy bars containing more than 500 calories eg Cadbury's Boost	"We believe warning labels may eventually be imposed with a negative effect for the category."
Ban/Tax on Unhealthy Products	"Moderate taxes may not necessarily lead to a decline in obesity rate but will probably help government to finance the costs of informing consumers and treating patients."

405. This analysis is restricted to the impact of possible regulation of the food industry, particularly that targeting so-called junk food manufacturers. It is interesting to note that labelling, which relies on giving consumers more of an informed choice, is seen as likely to have relatively little effect on volumes. Conversely, more draconian measures aimed at reducing the choices available, are seen as more likely to be effective.

406. This raises a question very much at the heart of the debate, and one that we explored throughout our inquiry: how much is obesity the responsibility of the individual making life-style choices; and how much is it the responsibility of Government? This is not simply a philosophical question. It has political ramifications. One reason it is very difficult for governments to intervene is that they risk criticism for operating a 'nanny-state', interfering in the lives of their citizens.

407. We fully accept that there is a degree to which obesity is the personal responsibility of individuals. This is clearly not so plausibly the case for children, who are usually deemed less able to make informed choices. Even here, however, we concede that parents do have a responsibility to try to feed their children healthily, though we acknowledge that, often, unhealthy food is cheaper than healthy options.

408. Whatever stance governments favour politically or philosophically they will inevitably have to deal with the consequences of the epidemic of obesity. If the very existence of the NHS in its present form is threatened by costs spiralling totally out of control it is hard to see that the Government will not, ultimately, be forced to intervene.

409. **Overall in our report we have looked for positive solutions. We have noted the example of Finland, where the force for change came from a grass-roots consumer response which took Government with it, rather than vice versa. We have at several junctures recommended voluntary agreements rather than regulation. We have chosen to accept the word of many representatives of the food industry that they wish to be part of the solution as well as part of the problem. Our belief is that this is a line worth pursuing, not only because it is politically far easier, but also because it could achieve results more quickly than a protracted battle to implement regulation.**

410. **Other pressures will be brought to bear on the food industry. Consumers may start to demand healthier products once unhealthy ones are properly labelled. Litigation— which is already happening in the USA—may alter the products available and customers' perception of those products. The greatly increased media attention to the problem of obesity may ripple through society and produce a change in behaviour.**

411. **This is an optimistic way of looking at the future. However, the recent past trends in the growth of obesity and overweight across the population must temper such optimism. Our concluding thought is that the Government must be prepared to act and intervene more forcefully and more directly if voluntary agreements fail. We recommend that the Government should allow three years to establish those areas where voluntary regulation and co-operation between the food industry and Government have worked and those where they have failed. It should then either extend the voluntary controls or introduce direct regulation.**

Conclusions and recommendations

1. The Clerk's Department Scrutiny Unit has recalculated the total estimated cost of obesity is £3.3–3.7 billion. This is £0.7–1.1 billion (27–42%) more than the NAO estimate for 1998. The difference between the two figures occurs for a number of reasons including higher NHS and drug costs, more accurate data that have been produced recently, the inclusion of more co-morbidities and the increased prevalence of obesity. This figure should still be regarded as an under-estimate. We note that these analyses are for the 20% of the adult population who are already obese. If in crude terms the costs of being overweight are on average only half of those of being obese then, with more than twice as many overweight as obese men and women, these costs would double. This would yield an overall cost estimate for overweight and obesity of £6.6–7.4 billion per year. (Paragraph 66)

2. Given the profound significance of overweight and obesity to the population we believe it is essential that the Government has access to accurate data on the actual calories the population is consuming, including figures for confectionery, soft drinks, alcohol and meals taken outside of the home. Although we acknowledge the difficulties of obtaining accurate data, given the limitations of any self-reported survey, the current information is very weak and clearly underestimates actual calorie consumption. We recommend that work is urgently commissioned to establish a Food Survey that accurately reflects the total calorie intake of the population to supersede the flawed and partial analysis currently available. The Food Standards Agency and Scientific Advisory Committee on Nutrition should advise on this. (Paragraph 72)

3. The relationship between alcohol consumption and obesity is too little understood. We recommend that the Department of Health commissions research into the correlation between trends in alcohol consumption and trends in obesity. (Paragraph 87)

4. We were appalled that a £710,000 campaign, launched by one of Britain's largest snack manufacturers, deliberately deployed a tactic which explicitly sought to undermine parental control over children's nutrition by exploiting children's natural tendency to attempt to influence their parents. The fact that this campaign was approved by the Advertising Standards Authority does not exonerate it, but merely demonstrates the ineffectiveness of current ASA standards and procedures. (Paragraph 111)

5. The causes of obesity are diverse, complex, and, in the main, underpinned by what are now entrenched societal norms. They are problems for which, as our expert witnesses have emphasised, no one simple solution exists. However, to fail to address this problem would be to condemn future generations, for the first time in over a century, to shorter life expectancies than their parents. A recent report by the Royal College of Physicians, Royal College of Paediatrics and Child Health, and the Faculty of Public Health emphasised the need for solutions to be "long term and sustainable, recognising that behaviour change is complex, difficult and takes time." We believe that an integrated and wide-ranging programme of solutions must be adopted as a

matter of urgency, and that the Government must show itself prepared to invest in the health of future generations by supporting measures which do not promise overnight results, but which constitute a consistent, effective and defined strategy. (Paragraph 153)

6. While the NHS is clearly central to tackling obesity through providing specialist health promotion and treatment for people who are already obese, we believe that the most important and dramatic changes will have to take place outside the doctor's surgery, in the wider environment in which people live their lives. And while we recognise that individuals have a key role to play in determining their own health and lifestyles, as the main factors contributing to the rapid rises in obesity seen in recent years are societal, it is critical that obesity is tackled first and foremost at a societal rather than an individual level. (Paragraph 154)

7. We feel strongly that the problem of obesity needs to be recognised and tackled at the highest levels across government. We therefore recommend that a specific Cabinet public health committee is appointed, chaired by the Secretary of State for Health, and that one of its first tasks is to oversee the development of Public Service Agreement (PSA) targets relating to public health in general and obesity in particular, across all relevant government departments. (Paragraph 159)

8. We recommend that the Government should consider either expanding the role of an existing body or bodies, such as the Food Standards Agency or Central Council of Physical Recreation (or linking these), or consider the creation of a new Council of Nutrition and Physical Activity to improve co-ordination and inject independent thinking into strategy. (Paragraph 160)

9. We strongly endorse the Wanless Report's recommendation that the Government must assign clear responsibility for the health educational role, previously played by the Health Education Authority, a fact made clear in correspondence from the Department to the Committee. (Paragraph 169)

10. We were very surprised that despite its occupying 'joint top priority' on the Government's public health agenda, there have been no health education campaigns aimed at tackling obesity. Although we acknowledge its benefits, we do not accept the Government's view that the Five-a-day fruit and vegetable promotion campaign is either designed for, or capable of, addressing the nutritional aspects of obesity. In recent years the Government has funded health education campaigns around, amongst other things, smoking, teenage pregnancy and sexually transmitted infections. The order in which other public health issues have been addressed, and the exclusion to date of obesity from this list, make the Government's actions in this area appear haphazard rather than strategic. (Paragraph 170)

11. If the Government intends seriously to address obesity through health promotion, it must adopt a health education campaign dedicated exclusively to tackling obesity, which should follow the model used in the recent anti-smoking campaign, plainly spelling out the health risks associated with being overweight or obese, and also highlighting those nutritional and lifestyle patterns which are most conducive to weight gain. It should specifically identify 'high risk' foods and drinks, and should

also emphasise the fact that consuming alcoholic drinks, like any other high-calorie food or drink, can also be conducive to unhealthy weight gain. At the same time, it should highlight the importance of physical activity both in preventing obesity and reducing weight levels. Part of the campaign should emphasise the crucial links between obesity and diabetes, and between obesity and cancer (which we have heard is barely known by the public as a whole). We recommend that such a health promotion campaign should be launched as soon as possible, with the Food Standards Agency advising on the nutritional content of such promotion, and the Activity Co-ordination Team, if this remains operational, or alternatively Sport England through its links with Move4Health advising on the physical activity dimension. (Paragraph 171)

12. Understanding the importance of healthy eating is meaningless without the skills to put these messages into practice. The huge demand for initiatives such as the Focus on Food Cooking Bus is a testimony to the extremely limited opportunities for cooking and food training within schools, and also to the desire of both pupils and teachers to have access to this type of training. While we fully support these initiatives and acknowledge the good work they are doing to bring this training back within reach of school pupils, we feel that learning about how to choose and prepare healthy meals should be an integral part of every young person's education, not an optional extra delivered only periodically. This is currently not the case. We recommend that the Government takes steps to reformulate the Food Technology curriculum, so that children of all ages receive practical training in how to choose and prepare healthy food which they can put into practice in their daily lives. As well as practical cookery lessons and classroom lessons about nutrition, children should also be taught how to understand food labelling and how to distinguish food advertising and marketing from objective fact; they could put their knowledge to the test in visits to a local supermarket. Healthy Schools initiatives have demonstrated the additional value of engaging children in projects to grow their own fruit and vegetables, fostering an understanding of where foods come from as well as reinforcing their motivation to eat more healthily. This should also form part of the food curriculum in schools. In order to achieve this, steps will need to be taken to strengthen teacher training in these areas. (Paragraph 174)

13. We recommend that delivery of the Food Technology curriculum should be rigorously inspected by Ofsted. (Paragraph 175)

14. Health promotion campaigns, as the recent anti-smoking advertising campaign has demonstrated, can play a successful role in raising awareness of the risks associated with particular behaviours, and to this end we have recommended that a health education campaign targeting obesity is launched as soon as possible. However, our evidence suggests that obesity has increased rapidly despite the fact that the benefits of a healthy diet have been well known for over 20 years. While we accept that individuals have the right and the responsibility to make choices about their own health and lifestyle, and we accept the importance of health education in enabling them to do so, we believe that to tackle obesity successfully education must be supported by a wider range of measures designed to remove the key barriers to choosing a healthy diet. We therefore recommend that the Government should concentrate its efforts not solely on informing choice, but also on addressing

environmental factors in order to, in its own words, make healthy choices easier to make. (Paragraph 181)

15. While we would clearly support an expansion in the promotion of healthy foods to redress the balance which currently lies entirely in favour of unhealthy foods, this alone seems to be an idealistic and ill thought-through notion, one which we are surprised that the Secretary of State for Culture, Media and Sport was prepared to espouse. (Paragraph 185)

16. Given the scale of the public health hazard the country is confronted by, it would seem appropriate to employ a precautionary approach where evidence is contradictory. As we have said previously, we are committed to long-term solutions to the problem of obesity. The Hastings Review offered stark evidence of the extent to which advertisers of less healthy foods were saturating broadcasting slots targeting children, who are often watching without any adult present. While we would not want to go so far as to call for an outright ban of all advertising of unhealthy food, given the clear evidence we have uncovered of the cynical exploitation of pester power we would very much welcome it if the industry as a whole acted in advance of any possible statutory control, and voluntarily withdrew such advertising. There is clear evidence that the majority of parents do not favour such advertisements during children's television. (Paragraph 192)

17. In one crucial sense, however, we share a concern about the effectiveness of banning or controlling television advertising: as noted above it is only a small part of the enormous food marketing effort that is aimed at children. If television advertising were to be banned, the marketing effort would simply be displaced to other areas— money previously spent on television advertising would, for example, be diverted to point of sale or internet promotion. (Paragraph 193)

18. We gather that the Secretary of State for Culture, Media and Sport is in discussion with OFCOM over the marketing of less healthy foods. We would like her to review the whole marketing function. In particular, we would like her to address some of the issues the Irish Broadcasting authorities are looking at, namely the impact of product endorsement of less healthy food by sports stars, and other celebrities; guidance on how these products can actually fit into a healthy diet, perhaps linking into nutritional information; and their impact on the energy equation in terms of the activity needed to displace the calories they add. Assuming the food and advertising industry is genuine in its desire to be part of the solution, a starting point for this would be for companies to agree clear public health targets. (Paragraph 194)

19. As we noted earlier, we were disturbed at the ineffectiveness of the Advertising Standards Authority, which is an industry self-regulation system. We recommend that OFCOM be asked to review the role of the ASA with a view to improving its effectiveness. This is not the first occasion on which the Health Committee has found the performance of the ASA to be disappointing. (Paragraph 195)

20. We feel that the school environment can have a strong influence over children's developing nutritional habits, and that the Government must not neglect this crucial opportunity to promote healthy eating to children and help them develop sound

lifelong habits. Healthy eating messages learnt through the national curriculum and Government healthy eating initiatives such as the schools fruit campaign will be contradicted and undermined if, within that same school environment, children are exposed to sponsorship messages from unhealthy food manufacturers, and given access to vending machines selling unhealthy products. There is evidence that parents are keen to see unhealthy influences removed from schools, with recent research finding that as many as 70% of parents were in favour of banning vending machines in schools. Recent research by the FSA also indicates that children are willing to purchase healthier drinks from vending machines when they are given the option. Given the worryingly steep rise in levels of childhood obesity, we feel that parents, teachers and school governors must all be fully engaged in tackling it, and that obesity should command a high priority on school board agendas. (Paragraph 199)

21. We therefore recommend that all schools should be required to develop school nutrition policies, in conjunction with parents and children, with the particular aim of combating obesity, but also of improving nutrition more generally. In conjunction with this, the Government should issue guidance to all schools strongly recommending that that they do not accept sponsorship from manufacturers associated with unhealthy foods or install vending machines selling unhealthy foods. If Government insists that this is a matter for local determination, we believe that governors should permit such practices only if these are shown to be supported by a clear majority of parents. The guidance should also give firm support for the replacement of existing vending machines with ones selling healthy foods and drinks. (Paragraph 200)

22. Nutritional labelling is intended to help consumers make sound nutritional decisions when buying food, but the current state of such labelling seems to be having, if anything, the opposite effect. We have repeatedly heard the argument, both from the food industry and from the Government, that there are no such things as good or bad foods, only good or bad diets. However, both the food industry and the Government have embraced the concept of labelling certain foods as 'healthy' with great enthusiasm, inviting the obvious conclusion that other foods must be, by definition, less healthy. (Paragraph 214)

23. The Government must accept the clear fact that some foods, which are extremely energy-dense, should only be eaten in moderation by most people, and we therefore recommend that it introduces legislation to effect a 'traffic light' system for labelling foods, either 'red—high', 'amber—medium' or 'green—low' according to criteria devised by the Food Standards Agency, which should be based on energy density. This would apply to all foods. Not only will such a system make it far easier for consumers to make easy choices, but it will also act as an incentive for the food industry to re-examine the content of their foods, to see if, for example, they could reduce fat or sugar to move their product from the 'high' category into the 'medium' category. (Paragraph 216)

24. Bearing in mind Derek Wanless's suggestion that greater effort needs to be made to measure the effectiveness of different interventions, we believe that this recommendation would lend itself well to objective assessment. If the scheme we

propose is accepted, it would be relatively simple to measure the impact on the range of relatively healthy and unhealthy foods offered by supermarkets, and any shift in the patterns of consumption from relatively unhealthy to relatively healthy products. (Paragraph 217)

25. We note the Government has made efforts to date to reduce salt levels in foods, but we feel that urgent attention should also be given towards tackling obesity. We recommend that, rather than targeting sugar and fat separately, the Government should focus on reducing the overall energy density of foods, and should work with the Food Standards Agency to develop stringent targets for reformulation of foods to reduce energy density within a short time frame. While we expect that reformulation could be achieved through voluntary arrangements with industry, and while we believe that the introduction of legislation in respect of labelling will encourage industry to make the entire product range healthier, the Government must be prepared, in the last resort, to underpin this with tougher measures in the near future if voluntary measures fail. (Paragraph 222)

26. The notion of taxing unhealthy foods is fraught with ideological and economic complexities, and at this stage we have not seen evidence that taking such a significant and difficult step would necessarily have the hoped-for effect of reducing obesity. We recommend, instead, that the Government should keep an open mind on this issue, and monitor closely the effect of fat taxes introduced in other countries. We also recommend that the Government should take steps to address the anomalies in the current arrangements for VAT on unhealthy 'treat' foods as it is clearly ludicrous that VAT is levied on ice cream and fizzy drinks but not on Bourbon biscuits or cakes. (Paragraph 228)

27. We hope that as the Government and food industry work together to reduce the energy density of foods, the need for 'healthy' options will be gradually reduced, with standard versions of foods being healthy as a matter of course. However, as this is likely to be a phased process, we recommend that in the short term the Government must work with the food industry to ensure that 'healthy' versions of foods, with reduced calories and fat, are available at an affordable price. (Paragraph 230)

28. As a matter of urgency, the Government must redouble its efforts to reform the Common Agricultural Policy as part of the public health agenda, and the future UK presidency from July 2005 will afford an opportunity for this to be done. Obesity is, after all, a growing problem in almost all EU countries. The issue of agricultural policy presents a perfect opportunity for the Government to demonstrate that it is committed to tackling public health issues in a joined-up way, an opportunity which in our view it has to date entirely neglected. However, as noted above, progress on the CAP will be extremely difficult unless public heath is given much greater emphasis in Europe. We therefore call on the Government to use its influence, and its forthcoming presidency, to encourage the Commission to reconsider the Treaty of Rome and put public health on an equal footing with trade and economics. (Paragraph 237)

29. In the interim, the Government, led by the Treasury should emulate the Swedish Government and produce a Health Audit of the CAP, and build a stronger alliance of

Health Ministries to combat other interests protecting the status quo in public policy. (Paragraph 238)

30. During this inquiry we have heard repeatedly that industry is keen to be 'part of the solution'. If this desire is to be translated into reality, then supermarkets should adopt new pro-active pricing strategies that positively support healthy eating, rather than acquiesce in the view that their duty to their customers goes no further than simply providing the range of foods which they want to buy. As part of their healthy pricing strategies, supermarkets must commit themselves to phasing out price promotions that favour unhealthy foods, and also stop all forms of product placement which give undue emphasis to unhealthy foods, in particular the placement of confectionery and snacks at supermarket checkouts. Alongside this, all sectors of the food industry should collaborate in the phasing out of super-sized food portions. We expect that the food industry will be keen to capitalise on the significant commercial opportunity that introducing these policies will present, and indeed much good work has already been done in this area. Several supermarkets have already committed themselves to banning the placement of confectionery at checkouts, and Kraft and McDonalds have begun to limit the availability of super-size portions. We commend fast-food outlets for offering fruit and salad options, though we request that these should be promoted more effectively than at present. Those companies who do not comply with Government guidance on healthy pricing, including product placement and super-sizing, should be publicly named and shamed. (Paragraph 241)

31. We recommend that the Department for Education and Skills extend the scope of the FSA review of the implementation of nutritional standards, with a view to developing appropriate nutrient based standards for school breakfasts. (Paragraph 248)

32. Furthermore, we recommend that the Department for Education and Skills takes steps to ensure that all children eat a healthy school meal at lunchtime, both through improving the provision of attractive and palatable 'healthy' options, and through restricting the availability of unhealthy foods. The Government should shift from the current 'food-based' standards towards the 'nutrition-based' standards being introduced in Scotland. The quality of school meals should also be taken into account by Ofsted inspections. (Paragraph 249)

33. We commend the wide range of measures and substantial funding being directed by the Government towards physical activity, particularly in schools. While we have reservations about the effectiveness of measures taken to date, we wish to pay tribute to the efforts that have been made in the last two years and to acknowledge the substantial funding that has been provided. (Paragraph 268)

34. We regard it as lamentable that the majority of the nation's youth are still not receiving two hours of sport and physical activity per week. While we very much welcome the DCMS/DfES target to have 75% of school children thus active by 2006 we do not believe that this goes far enough. We have reservations about the quality of much of the activity undertaken, since little work has been done to establish what the two hours involves, and whether it includes, for example, time taken in travelling to

and from facilities. Moreover, even the two hour target puts England below the EU average in terms of physical activity in school, despite the fact that childhood obesity is accelerating more quickly here than elsewhere. (Paragraph 275)

35. We recommend that, given the threat of obesity to the current generation of children and taking account of the proven contribution of physical activity to academic achievement, the aspiration should be for school children to participate in three hours per week of physical activity, as recommended by the European Heart Network. (Paragraph 276)

36. Relentless pressure on the curriculum has served to squeeze out school sport and PE. However, there is ample evidence that being physically active benefits children's academic performance, and many schools in the independent sector offer four or more hours of exercise per week. We know that the Government is monitoring closely the Brent project but that it has been less than forthcoming with supportive funding. We believe that this is a fascinating pilot project and would like to see it rigorously evaluated. Given its potential importance as a model, we also think it would be helpful if the Department's favourable initial appraisal of the scheme were supported by funding. (Paragraph 277)

37. We recommend that the Curriculum Authority should address ways of diversifying organised and recreational activity in schools to embrace areas such as dance or aerobics to broaden the appeal of PE and to counteract the elitism, embarrassment and bullying that the changing room sometimes creates. (Paragraph 278)

38. We do not think it appropriate that the activity of a school in delivering the physical activity agenda should be extrinsic to any evaluation of its overall performance. Physical activity is not—or should not be—a second order consideration. Not only is it crucial to children's health but it also directly benefits academic performance. So we recommend that the Ofsted inspection criteria should be extended to include a school's performance in encouraging and sustaining physical activity. (Paragraph 279)

39. We recommend that the Department for Education and Skills, as part of its wider work to improve self-esteem and self-confidence amongst school children, should ensure that each school, as part of its policy against bullying, remains alert to the particular issue of bullying of children who are overweight or obese. Teachers should receive training in children's diet, physical activity levels, and how to help obese children combat bullying, without further stigmatising them. (Paragraph 280)

40. We believe that providing safe routes to school for walking and cycling, adequate and safe play areas in and out of school is very important in the battle against obesity. (Paragraph 284)

41. The measures proposed by the Environment, Transport and Regional Affairs Committee in its report *Walking in Towns* 2001 strike us as sensible and persuasive and we are sorry so little action has been taken to implement them. (Paragraph 287)

42. Given the profound impact increased levels of activity would have on the nation's health, quite aside from the obvious environmental benefits, it seems to us entirely

unacceptable that successive governments have been so remiss in effectively promoting active travel. (Paragraph 288)

43. We regard the failure of the Department for Transport to produce a National Walking Strategy over a period of almost ten years as scandalous. This very inactivity clearly demonstrates that the priorities of the Department lie elsewhere. We would be extremely disappointed if concerns about political embarrassment had indeed obstructed such an important policy. One way of defusing any political embarrassment would be to incorporate the walking strategy into a wider anti-obesity strategy. (Paragraph 292)

44. We believe it would be helpful if commercial firms issuing pedometers also issued guidance agreed with Sport England and the FSA, on the recommended activity levels per day and on the correlation between steps taken and calories consumed. (Paragraph 297)

45. We welcome the funding the Department of Health has provided to a pilot project on the use of pedometers. We recommend that the Department co-ordinates inter-departmental activity with a view to achieving wide-spread use of pedometers in schools, the workplace and the wider community. (Paragraph 299)

46. It would not be appropriate for us to spell out the individual measures required to achieve the Government's ambitious cycling targets, although we were particularly impressed by the segregation of cyclists from road traffic we witnessed in Odense. If the Government were to achieve its target of trebling cycling in the period 2000–2010 (and there are very few signs that it will) that might achieve more in the fight against obesity than any individual measure we recommend within this report. So we would like the Department of Health to have a strategic input into transport policy and we believe it would be an important symbolic gesture of the move from a sickness to a health service if the Department of Health offered funding to support the Department for Transport's sustainable transport town pilots. (Paragraph 316)

47. There will be profound economic as well as health costs to be paid if the current obesity epidemic continues unchecked. Major planning proposals and transport projects are already subject to environmental impact assessment; we believe that it would be appropriate if a health impact assessment were also a statutory requirement. This would enable health to be integrated into the planning procedure and help bring about the sort of creative, joined-up solution which is required. This may seem a cumbersome and drastic step but we believe that only such strong measures will help reverse the dramatic decline in everyday activity that has occurred in recent decades. (Paragraph 321)

48. We recommend that the Department of Health, in conjunction with the Department for Work and Pensions and the Department of Trade and Industry first organises a major conference to promote awareness of obesity in the work-place and then engages in an ongoing process of consultation to see how measures can be taken to address sedentary behaviour. We recommend that these Departments consult with the Treasury to see what fiscal incentives can be provided to promote active travel. (Paragraph 328)

49.   We also recommend that the public sector looks to set an example in finding creative ways of encouraging activity in everyday life, and that this is built into a PSA target for each Department. (Paragraph 329)

50.   We welcome the creation of the Activity Co-ordination Team though we regret it took so long for it to begin its work. Anything that co-ordinates Government activity in this complex and challenging field is worthwhile. We await with interest the publication of its first report. We recommend that its reports explicitly link its activity to the Government's specific targets on activity both in schools and in the community. (Paragraph 334)

51.   The Department agreed that Strategic Health Authorities (SHAs) should have information about local work on obesity at their fingertips, and we recommend that a survey of action on obesity, both at PCT and SHA level, should be undertaken as part of the ongoing work on the forthcoming White Paper on public health. (Paragraph 337)

52.   We feel strongly that Primary Care Trusts should be taking a more active role in preventing obesity, and urge the Government to ensure that PCTs have the capacity, competency and incentive to fulfil their crucial obligation to safeguard the public health of the local communities they serve. We also endorse the recommendation of the Wanless report that the Healthcare Commission should develop a robust mechanism for assessing performance of both PCTs and Strategic Health Authorities with respect to public health. (Paragraph 343)

53.   We feel that this country's well developed network of primary care providers, local GPs, provides a unique resource for health promotion and for the identification and management of patients who are overweight or obese. However, managing weight problems sensitively and successfully requires specialist skills, and we are concerned by suggestions that obesity is viewed by many clinicians as a lifestyle issue rather than a serious health problem requiring active management to prevent dire health consequences. We deplore the low priority given to obesity by the new GP contract. We hope that NICE guidance on the prevention, identification, evaluation, treatment and weight maintenance of overweight and obesity, currently expected in Summer 2006, will go some way towards increasing the priority of obesity within general practice, as well as helping primary care practitioners develop and improve the services they provide in this difficult area. The Government should also ensure that within each PCT area there is at least one specialist primary care obesity clinic, probably supported by a range of different health professionals, to which GPs can refer any patients they identify as needing specialist support to address a developing or existing weight problem. (Paragraph 355)

54.   We recommend that, in establishing primary care obesity clinics, PCTs should fully explore the possibilities of using less traditional models of service delivery, involving clinicians from across the professional spectrum, from nurses to pharmacists to dieticians. The full range of interventions available to treat obesity includes diet, lifestyle, medical treatment and surgical treatment. (Paragraph 356)

55. We also took some interesting evidence from commercial slimming organisations. We recommend that the NHS examines whether their expertise can be brought to bear in devising strategies to combat obesity holistically. (Paragraph 357)

56. Obesity is a serious medical problem. Although in common with other illnesses, its prevention and some first-line management can be delivered within a primary care setting, patients with more entrenched or complex problems need prompt access to specialist medical care. Childhood obesity is a worrying and increasingly common subset of this illness, and children in particular need specialist care. Yet specialist obesity services seem to be an almost entirely neglected area of the NHS, apparently exempt from Government initiatives to push down waiting times despite their obvious importance in preventing a large range of other debilitating and costly diseases. We therefore recommend that the Government provides funding for the large scale expansion of obesity services in secondary care, underpinned by careful management to ensure that the service provision is matched to need. The Government's maximum waiting time targets must apply to all of these services. (Paragraph 363)

57. We were appalled to learn of the desperate inadequacy of treatment and support services for obese children. Steps must be taken to ensure that obese children and young people have prompt access to specialist treatment wherever they live. (Paragraph 366)

58. We recommend that throughout their time at school, children should have their Body Mass Index measured annually at school, perhaps by the school nurse, a health visitor, or other appropriate health professional. The results should be sent home in confidence to their parents, together with, where appropriate, advice on lifestyle, follow-up, and referral to more specialised services. Where appropriate, BMI measurement could be carried out alongside other health care interventions which are delivered at school, for example inoculation programmes. Care will need to be taken to avoid stigmatising children who are overweight or obese, but given that research indicates that many parents are no longer even able to identify whether their children are overweight or not, this seems to us a vital step in tackling obesity. (Paragraph 369)

59. We were dismayed to hear that a specialist GP who devoted much of his time to trying to tackle obesity in his local population was being put under pressure from his local PCT to reduce his prescribing of drugs to tackle obesity, despite these drugs having received approval from NICE, with the corresponding obligation on PCTs to provide funding for them. We were told by the same doctor that in 15 years of practice he had never received communications questioning his prescribing rates for drugs to treat heart disease or diabetes, two illnesses frequently caused by obesity. This provides a telling exposé of current attitudes towards obesity, whereby it is regarded by NHS decision-makers as a lifestyle problem for which treatment is an optional extra. We recommend that the Government takes urgent steps to tackle this subtle deprioritisation of obesity wherever it occurs in the NHS. (Paragraph 372)

60. Bariatric surgery is in no way a panacea for the current obesity epidemic. Rather it is a high-risk, invasive surgical procedure that represents a last line of defence for

people with life-threatening morbid obesity. However as the number of people suffering from morbid obesity in England looks set to increase, it is an option that needs to be made available to all those who need it, and it is unacceptable that in some parts of the UK patients with a life-threatening condition are having to wait as long as four years for bariatric surgery. We hope that the measures we have recommended to improve provision of specialist obesity services in both primary and secondary care will help to address the problem that many patients are not referred for bariatric surgery simply because their local doctors are not aware that it is an option. However, the NHS needs also to ensure that adequate service capacity is in place fully to meet need, which is patently not the case at present. The Government must devote protected resources to ensuring that bariatric surgery is available to all those who need it, and should issue guidelines for the strategic development of services across the country, to eliminate the current postcode provision of obesity surgery. (Paragraph 379)

61. We feel it is vital that advances in medical and surgical treatment of obesity should be supported by equivalent development of services to address the psychological and behavioural aspects of obesity. All those receiving treatment for obesity, whether in a primary or in secondary care setting, should have access to psychological support provided by an appropriate professional, whether this is a psychiatrist, psychologist, psychotherapist, counsellor, or family therapist. (Paragraph 382)

62. The evidence we received during the course of this inquiry has convinced us that despite its overwhelming importance, obesity remains a low priority for the majority of service commissioners and providers in the NHS. The National Health Service has a responsibility both to take strategic action to prevent obesity, as part of its public health remit, and to provide adequate treatment for those already suffering from overweight or obesity, as it would for those suffering from any other medical condition. It appears to us to be failing in both of these areas, and this needs to change as a matter of urgency. (Paragraph 393)

63. We are fully aware that obesity is mentioned in existing NSFs, but we believe that these scant mentions are woefully inadequate to provide a strategic framework through which to tackle what has been described as 'the biggest public health threat of the twenty-first century'. We also understand that a public health White Paper will be published in the summer, but again we fear that the extent and seriousness of the obesity problem will be lost by including obesity only as part of a wider umbrella of general public health initiatives. (Paragraph 394)

64. We note the Government's reservations about committing to further National Service Frameworks, which they voiced in response to our report on *Sexual Health*. However, the current structure of the National Service Framework programme places too great an emphasis on tackling discrete disease areas, focusing on downstream consequences at the expense of the upstream contributors to these diseases, including obesity. Indeed, we heard compelling evidence that many general practices are unable to devote time to tackling obesity because of their obligation to meet targets in the Coronary Heart Disease and Diabetes NSFs, even though, ironically, many of these 'competing' disease areas can be directly improved by tackling obesity. And while it is clear that general public health problems, such as

smoking, can be addressed within disease-based NSFs, the lack of obesity targets has led to this area being systematically neglected. (Paragraph 395)

65. It is essential that, as part of the Government's wider strategy to tackle obesity, a dedicated framework document is produced to emphasise to a largely sceptical NHS the full scale and seriousness of this problem. The complexity of the challenge facing the NHS in this area, including the need to develop services and care pathways across all tiers of service delivery in a rapidly changing area of medicine, as well as to take the lead on prevention and health promotion, makes a detailed strategic framework vital. This document should build on existing work in this area, drawing together and emphasising the obesity measures already set out in the National Service Frameworks, and linking in with the ongoing work of NICE. Crucially, it must re-introduce realistic but stretching targets for reducing the prevalence of obesity and overweight over the next ten years, underpinned by more detailed, service-based targets, in particular bringing waiting times for specialist medical and surgical obesity services in line with all other NHS specialties. PCTs should be stringently performance-managed on their delivery of these targets. (Paragraph 396)

66. It would be very difficult to disaggregate the possible impact of any of the recommendations we make. We have argued for a coherent package of measures, addressing both sides of the energy equation. We believe they would have more chance of being effective if implemented in full rather than in a piecemeal fashion. However, it is clearly important that some steps are taken to monitor the effectiveness, and the cost-effectiveness of what we propose, in line with the recommendations of the Wanless report on public health. The National Audit Office undertook an influential and ground-breaking report on obesity in 2001. We know that they have maintained an interest in the subject thereafter. So we would like the National Audit Office to conduct further work on the value for money implications of measures taken to combat obesity, since this will be one of the greatest pressures on NHS resources over the coming decades. In calling for this, we also note the point made in the Scrutiny Unit analysis annexed to our report that there is a "severe lack" of official estimates of the costs of diseases relating to obesity. We recommend that the Department undertakes urgent work to establish better estimates of the cost of treating diseases to allow it to manage its resources more effectively. (Paragraph 403)

67. Overall in our report we have looked for positive solutions. We have noted the example of Finland, where the force for change came from a grass-roots consumer response which took Government with it, rather than vice versa. We have at several junctures recommended voluntary agreements rather than regulation. We have chosen to accept the word of many representatives of the food industry that they wish to be part of the solution as well as part of the problem. Our belief is that this is a line worth pursuing, not only because it is politically far easier, but also because it could achieve results more quickly than a protracted battle to implement regulation. (Paragraph 409)

68. Other pressures will be brought to bear on the food industry. Consumers may start to demand healthier products once unhealthy ones are properly labelled. Litigation—which is already happening in the USA—may alter the products available and customers' perception of those products. The greatly increased media attention to

the problem of obesity may ripple through society and produce a change in behaviour. (Paragraph 410)

69. This is an optimistic way of looking at the future. However, the recent past trends in the growth of obesity and overweight across the population must temper such optimism. Our concluding thought is that the Government must be prepared to act and intervene more forcefully and more directly if voluntary agreements fail. We recommend that the Government should allow three years to establish those areas where voluntary regulation and co-operation between the food industry and Government have worked and those where they have failed. It should then either extend the voluntary controls or introduce direct regulation. (Paragraph 411)

Annex 1: The economic costs of obesity: A note prepared by the Scrutiny Unit, Clerk's Department, House of Commons

1. This annex sets out to give a broad estimate of the cost of obesity in England. It uses the methodology employed by the NAO in *Tackling Obesity in England*. It updates the data used in that report, from 1998 figures to the latest available, which is 2002 in most cases. It extends the coverage of the calculations to look at a wider range of diseases that are attributable to obesity. It looks at future costs in a very general way. It makes no specific cost estimates, but identifies the driving forces and how increases in costs might differ from increases in the prevalence of obesity.

NAO report

2. *Tackling Obesity in England* estimated that the direct cost of treating obesity and its consequences was £480 million (1.5% of NHS expenditure) and indirect costs (loss of earnings due to sickness and premature mortality) amounted to £2.1 billion. Both figures relate to 1998. A total projected figure of £3.6 billion was given for 2010. On numerous occasions the authors state that they believe various elements to either be conservative estimates or underestimates, due to the exclusion of a number of elements or a lack of data in certain areas:[1]

> We have deliberately produced conservative estimates to raise their credibility as the basis of further discussion of this report in the face of a number of uncertainties.

3. Some of the more expensive areas that were not included (for various reasons) include social care, lipid regulating drugs, appointments with primary care practitioners other than GPs, and the costs of depression and lower back pain attributable to obesity. The report's estimate was a point figure, rather than a range. Presumably this figure would have been at the bottom of any range estimate that would have been given.

4. *Tackling Obesity in England* mentioned that estimates of the direct costs of treating obesity from other countries with similar levels of obesity varied from 2–6% of health spending. If such a range applied to England then the costs would have been between £0.7 and £2.1 billion in 1998. The NAO figure was therefore lower than any of these 'comparable' countries. The table below summarises cost estimates for all countries alongside data on obesity levels. It shows the percentage cost figure for England at joint lowest with France. At the time of the estimates the rate of obesity in France was around one-third of the level in England, of the countries shown only the US had a higher level. The table only gives two recent estimates for the US. Studies from the mid-1980s to the mid 1990s gave a range of 5.5–7.8%.[2]

---

1   NAO, *Tackling Obesity in* England (2001), para. 2.27; see also appendix 6 paras 17-18, 22, 25, 28 and 33-34

2   *Obesity in Europe The Case for Action*, International Obesity Taskforce

Estimates of the direct costs of obesity

Country	Year of estimate	Proportion of total healthcare expenditure due to obesity	Prevalence of obesity (BMI>30)	
			At time of estimate	Latest
US	1999	8.5%	30.5%	30.5%
US	2000	4.8%	30.5%	30.5%
Netherlands	1981-89	4%	5.0%	10.3%
Canada	1997	2.4%	14.0%	13.9%
Portugal	1996	3.5%	11.5%	14.0%
Australia	1989/90	>2%	10.8%	22.0%
England	1998	1.5%	19.0%	23.5%
France	1992	1.5%	6.5%	9.0%

Sources: *Obesity in Europe The Case for Action, International Obesity Taskforce*

Wolf AM, Colditz GA. Current estimates of the economic cost of obesity in the United States. Obes Res. 1998 Mar; 6(2):97-106

The Surgeon General's Call to Action to Prevent and Decrease Overweight and Obesity, Office of the Surgeon General

Costs of Obesity, American Obesity Association

OECD Health Data 2003

5. Overall the table shows a wider range of estimates but an inconsistent link between higher obesity and higher costs. If we ignore England then at the extremes more obesity means a higher cost estimate and *vice versa*, but the picture is more mixed for the other countries. Given the very different use of cost estimation methods, definitions of obesity, population structures and systems of healthcare it would be remarkable if there were a simple linear relationship. It is highly likely that the very large range shown is in part due to differing methodologies and is presumably the most likely reason why the figure for England is where it is. It is particularly noticeable that only the US has multiple estimates (six since 1986). These have varied considerably. Having a range of estimates can improve the debate about the economic impacts of obesity.

6. There are even fewer estimates of the indirect costs of obesity from other countries. A study in the US estimated the indirect costs at slightly less than the direct costs ($47.6 billion, compared to $51.2 billion in 1995, uprated to $61 billion and $56 billion in 2000).[3] It is difficult to make any direct comparisons with the estimates for England, but the most striking difference is that indirect costs were smaller in the US estimate, but were over four times greater in the estimate for England.

Direct costs

Treating obesity

7. As mentioned earlier, the same basic methodology employed by the NAO is used for these calculations. The limitations outlined in *Tackling Obesity in England* should therefore be borne in mind when interpreting all the estimates in this Annex. There are some improved data sources that have recently become available, most notably *NHS Reference Costs* which give much more detailed and accurate cost information for different diagnosis/procedure groups.

---

3   Wolf AM, Colditz GA. "Current estimates of the economic cost of obesity in the United States", *Obesity Research* 1998 Mar; 6(2):97-106; *The Surgeon General's Call to Action to Prevent and Decrease Overweight and Obesity*, Office of the Surgeon General

8. *GP consultations* —The unit cost figure for GP consultations used here is from the same source as the NAO figure,[4] but also includes an element for direct care staff. As with the NAO figure there is no direct estimate of the costs of other primary practitioners. There is also no more up to date information on consultations for obesity. The 1991–92 figures are still the most up to date and comprehensive consultation rates.[5] Assuming that the number of consultations has increased in line with the prevalence of obesity[6] then costs would be in the region of £12–15 million. While simply increasing consultation figures by the percentage increase in obesity is a crude method, the alternative is to simply ignore the 50% increase in obesity since 1991–92.

9. *Ordinary admissions*—Using data on admissions for 2002–03[7] and the latest cost figures[8] gives an estimate of around £2 million. The actual number of admissions for obesity fell by almost 25% between 1998 and 2002.

10. *Day cases*—The number of day cases has increased slightly, but they are still very small in number at 360 in 2001–02. The estimated cost is £0.12 million.

11. *Outpatient attendances*—The number of outpatient attendances are uprated in the same way as GP consultations. Combined with a slightly higher unit cost the estimate is £0.5–0.7 million.

12. *Prescriptions*—The total cost for all obesity-related drugs has increased rapidly since 1998 with the licensing of orlistat. The total cost in 2002 was £31.3 million.[9] The chart below illustrates the pace of growth. Over the same period the number of prescriptions for orlistat increased from 18,000 to over 540,000. This may have resulted in a greater increase in GP consultation than that assumed earlier.

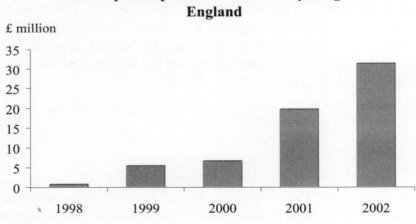

Cost of prescriptions for anti-obesity drugs in England

4   *Unit costs of health and social care 2003*, PSSRU, University of Kent at Canterbury

5   Morbidity Statistics from General Practice, fourth national study 1991-1992, MB5 no.3, RCGP/OPCS

6   Health Survey for England, 2002, DH (Department of Health)

7   Hospital Episode Statistics 2002-03, DH

8   NHS Reference Costs 2002, DH

9   Prescription Cost Analysis 2002, DH

13. When combined this gives a total estimated cost for treatment of between £46 million and £49 million. This is around four times the NAO figure, the vast majority of this increase being due to the increase in drug costs. The breakdown of this estimate and that produced by the NAO are given below.

The estimated costs of treating obesity in England: 1998 and 2002
£ millions

	1998	2002
GP consultations	6.8	12-15
Ordinary admissions	1.3	1.9
Day cases	0.1	0.1
Outpatient attendances	0.5	0.5-0.7
Prescriptions	0.8	31.3
Total cost of treating obesity	**9.5**	**45.8-49.0**

14. The real level of uncertainty is somewhat greater than that indicated in the table as the unit costs chosen are necessarily somewhat inexact. However, the most precise information is produced for prescription costs, the largest element, so there is a relatively small amount of uncertainty about this estimate.

Treating the consequences of obesity

15. The box opposite lists diseases and complications that are most often linked to obesity.[10] Those in bold were included and costed by the NAO. A number of the others were explicitly excluded. Just because a particular disease or condition has been linked in publications relating to obesity does not necessarily mean that there is research showing a significantly higher risk. In some cases the evidence is rather weak, mixed or absent. In others the diseases/conditions are far too unspecific to quantify, like 'reproductive problems' or 'surgical problems'. The evidence for these is more anecdotal.

16. Among the diseases not included by the NAO evidence of a statistically significant increased risk was found for post menopausal breast cancer,[11] lower back pain (among women only),[12] hyperlipidaemia[13] and sleep apnoea.[14] Of the remaining diseases/conditions depression has the greatest potential for altering any estimate of the cost of obesity.

17. The methodology for calculating total costs of these diseases is the same as that used for obesity. New estimates of the percentage of cases attributable to obesity were calculated for the additional diseases and updated for the original ones to take account of the increased prevalence of obesity between 1998 and 2002. Some further comments specific to these diseases are given below.

Diseases linked to obesity
Type 2 diabetes
Hypertension
Angina pectoris
Myocardial infarction
Cancers
Endometrial
Colon
Rectal
Ovarian
Prostate
Breast
Kidney
Gallbladder
Osteoarthritis
Gout
Stroke
Gallstones
End stage renal disease
Liver disease
Low back pain
Sleep apnoea
Urinary incontinence
Hyperlipidaemia
Polycystic Ovary Syndrome
Breathing problems
Complications in pregnancy
Complications in surgery
Psychological and social problems
Reproductive disorders

18. The following table shows estimates of the costs of treating the consequences of obesity for 2002 and compares this to the original estimates. Each element, and the total, is given a range to reflect the remaining uncertainty about the precise number of cases attributable to obesity.

10 This list is based on diseases associated with obesity in: Annual Report of the Chief Medical Officer 2002, Department of Health, American Obesity Association, Clinical Guidelines on the Identification, Evaluation and Treatment of Overweight and Obesity in Adults –The Evidence Report, National Institute of Health.

11 van den Brandt PA et al, "Pooled analysis of prospective cohort studies on height, weight and breast cancer risk", *Am J Epidemiol.* 2000 Sep 15; 152(6):514-27

12 Lake JK et al, "Back pain and obesity in the 1958 British birth cohort. Cause or effect?" *J Clin Epimemiol,* 2000 Mar 1;53(3):245-50

13 Brown CD et al, "Body mass index and the prevalence of hypertension and dyslipidaemia", *Obes Res.* 2000 Dec;8(9):605-19

14 Young T et al, "The occurrence of sleep-disordered breathing among middle-aged adults", *N Engl J Med.* 1993 Apr 29;328(17):1230-35

The estimated costs of treating the consequences of obesity in England: 1998 and 2002

£ millions

	1998	2002
GP consultations	45	90-105
Ordinary admissions	121	210-250
Day cases	5	10-15
Outpatient attendances	52	60-90
Prescriptions	247	575-625
Total cost of treating the consequences	**470**	**945-1,075**

19. The largest increase in percentage terms was in the cost of day cases; however at £5–10 million the actual increase was relatively small. The largest increase in cash terms was in the cost of prescriptions at around £225–275 million. The cost of outpatient attendances increased by the smallest proportion. Within individual diseases hypertension was still the most costly with a total of £225–275 million estimated as attributable to obesity. The next most costly was one of the additional co-morbidities added for this exercise—hyperlipidaemia. Its total attributable cost is estimated at £170–190 million, virtually all due to the cost of lipid-regulating drugs. This group is dominated by the statins—the National Service Framework on Coronary Heart Disease recommended their use and the total cost of such drugs dispensed increased more than three-fold between 1998 and 2002. They are now the most expensive drug group and their total cost is increasing at the fastest rate.[15]

20. In total the additional co-morbidities accounted for just over 20% of this estimate or £200–225 million. This is equivalent to around 40% of the difference between this estimate and the one in *Tackling Obesity in England*. The greater prevalence of obesity between 1998 and 2002 accounted for 12% of this difference and increased drug costs, take-up and availability a further 20%. It is not possible to say how much of the remaining increase was due other factors, like higher NHS costs or improved data.

21. Data from the 12 months to June 2003 show continuing significant increases in the cost of the drug groups that contribute most to the estimates above. Lipid-regulating drugs, anti-hypertensive therapy and drugs used in diabetes saw the three largest increases in total costs, up a combined 23%, or just under £300 million.[16] The implication of this for the costs of obesity is that the main element of expenditure is still increasing at a rapid pace, well above what might be expected from increases in the prevalence of these diseases alone.

All direct costs

22. The estimates in the previous two sections combine to give a total range for the direct costs of treating obesity and its consequences of £990–1,225 million (2.3–2.6% of net NHS expenditure in 2001–02), more than double the figure for 1998 given in *Tackling Obesity in*

15 Prescription Cost Analysis 2002, DH

16 Chief Executive's Report to the NHS 2002: Statistical Supplement, DH

England. All the limitations of that estimate apply to the updated version, specifically the exclusion of any social care data, incomplete data on primary care, reliance on international data on relative risk and the approximate nature of unit costs. All these must be considered when drawing any conclusions from these estimates. The lack of cost data in certain important areas and the number of associated diseases that have not been included means that these figures are still likely to underestimate the true cost of treating obesity and its consequences.

Indirect costs

Mortality

23. There is no need to include additional co-morbidities in the cost estimate for years of life lost as the NAO estimate used research that covered mortality from all causes. Applying the latest data on obesity rates by age and sex gives a figure of 34,100 deaths and around 45,000 attributable years of working life lost; an increase of 13% on the 1998 figures. Applying 2002 data on earnings[17] gives a total estimated cost due to premature mortality of £1.05–1.15 billion. This is an increase of around 20% on the 1998 figure from *Tackling Obesity in England.* This effect of higher wages and employment figures is broadly the same as the increased number of deaths resulting from higher obesity levels.

24. The overall number equates to 6.8% of deaths in England. While this is a significant number the World Health Organisation estimates that in developed countries 9.6% of deaths among men and 11.5% among women are due to overweight *and* obesity.[18] Applying these rates to deaths in England in 2001 gives a total of 52,500.[19]

Morbidity

25. Incapacity Benefit data was obtained from the Department for Work and Pensions on claimants with obesity and the other co-morbidities. This implied that there were 15.5–16 million attributable days of certified incapacity. This is equivalent to lost earnings of £1.3–1.45 billion—used as a proxy for production losses under the "human capital" approach. The range of this estimate goes from £20 million *less* than the 1998 figure to £130 million above. The estimated number of attributable days of incapacity is more than 10% below the estimate given for 1998, despite the inclusion of additional co-morbidities. Between 1998 and 2002 average daily earnings increased by 17.5%. The additional co-morbidities accounted for £190–210 million of this increase. The vast majority of this was for back pain. The relative risk of obese people developing back pain is quite small and only statistically significant for women. In these calculations only 5% of days of certified incapacity for lower back pain were attributable to obesity.

26. As indicated in *Tackling Obesity in England* the number of days of sickness attributable to obesity is an underestimate as it excludes self-certified days of sickness. This is counter-

---

17   Male and female average earnings in England adjusted for the national proportions of part-time working. *New Earnings Survey 2002*, ONS

18   The World Health Report 2002, WHO, table 4.9

19   Key population and vital statistics 2001, ONS

balanced by the fact that the obese group earns less than the national average wage figure used. It is not possible to say which of these factors is more important.

Conclusion

27. The following table combines all the estimates for 2002 and compares them to the 1998 figure. Overall this paper estimates that the cost of obesity in England was £3.3–3.7 billion in 2002. This is 27–42% above the figure given in *Tackling Obesity in England*; the midpoint is similar to its projection for 2010. It has been mentioned a number of times that a significant part of this increase is due to the inclusion of new co-morbidities in this analysis. An estimated £390–435 million of the increase was due to this. The remaining increase was due to a combination of increased drug costs, take-up and availability, improved data, higher NHS costs and higher earnings (in the economy as a whole) as well as an increase in the number of people who are obese. As has been indicated earlier, this total figure should still be seen as an underestimate.

The estimated cost of obesity in England: 1998 and 2002
£ millions

	1998 (NAO)	2002
GP consultations	6.8	12-15
Ordinary admissions	1.3	1.9
Day cases	0.1	.1
Outpatient attendances	0.5	0.5-0.7
Prescriptions	0.8	13.3
Total cost of treating obesity	**9.5**	**45.8-49.0**
GP consultations	44.9	90-105
Ordinary admissions	120.7	210-250
Day cases	5.2	10-15
Outpatient attendances	51.9	60-90
Prescriptions	247.2	575-625
Total cost of treating the consequences of obesity	**469.9**	**945-1,075**
Lost earnings due to attributable mortality	827.8	1,050-1,150
Lost earnings due to attributable sickness	1,321.7	1,300-1,450
Total indirect costs	**2,149.5**	**2,350-2,600**
Total cost of obesity	**2,628.9**	**3,340-3,724**

28. While this figure seems very large what does it really mean? Is it really that large? Some estimates for individual diseases are much higher. It is thought that diabetes and its co-morbidities consumes 9–10% of total NHS resources. The total (direct and indirect) costs of coronary heart disease and back pain have recently been estimated at £7.1 billion and £6.8 billion respectively.[20] Applying the method used in this paper the total cost of sickness absence due to depression is over £9 billion. The cost of smoking to the NHS in England was estimated at £1.4–1.7 billion in the mid-1990s, 4.3–5.3% of net spending.[21] In

---

20   Costs of selected diseases, 1999, UK www.heartstats.org

21   *Smoking Kills – White Paper on Tobacco* (Cm 4177); Department of Health Departmental Annual Report, various years.

this context the cost of obesity looks somewhat less significant. However, it is important to consider the rapid increase in obesity over the past two decades and the possibility that this might continue. The estimates of premature mortality due to obesity are significant in any context.

The future

29. This note only looks at future costs in a very general way. It is clear that, disregarding the additional co-morbidities, that changes in costs are not necessarily equal to changes in the prevalence of obesity. This is true even after general NHS inflation is accounted for. Other factors like new drugs, treatments and guidelines can radically increase costs. It is impossible to predict how these might alter the situation over the next decade. In addition to this there are further complicating factors. There is clearly a time lag between the onset of obesity and increases in related chronic diseases.[22] This suggests that further increases in health problems and economic costs are already 'locked in' and will increase. Similarly obesity can lead to diseases/conditions which are permanent—like gout and diabetes—while losing weight may help with their management health and cost implications remain. The rise in childhood obesity is likely to further multiply such effects as their exposure to risk is increased over a longer period.

Research and data

30. Data on relative risks of the associated diseases are largely international. This increases the uncertainty in cost estimates, especially when they are so reliant on the consequences of obesity. More research using data from the UK would improve the accuracy and credibility of such estimates. The methodology used for estimating costs is the best possible considering the available data, but it is not ideal. A number of simplifying assumptions have had to be made and methodologies vary for different types of costs. There is a severe lack of recent Department of Health/NHS estimates of the total costs of individual diseases/conditions. Some official estimates of the costs of the most important/expensive diseases and conditions would improve the public debate in this area and allow the burdens of a wide range to be put into a meaningful context.

Annex 2: Calculate your Body Mass Index

Body Mass Index Chart (English and Metric)[23]

To use find the intersection of your weight and height—this is your BMI.

Height (feet and inches)

Weight (pounds)	5'0"	5'1"	5'2"	5'3"	5'4"	5'5"	5'6"	5'7"	5'8"	5'9"	5'10"	5'11"	6'0"	6'1"	6'2"	6'3"	6'4"	Weight (kilograms)
100	20	19	18	18	17	17	16	16	15	15	14	14	14	13	13	12	12	45
105	21	20	19	19	18	17	17	16	16	16	15	15	14	14	13	13	13	47
110	21	21	20	19	19	18	18	17	17	16	16	15	15	15	14	14	13	50
115	22	22	21	20	20	19	19	18	17	17	17	16	16	15	15	14	14	52
120	23	23	22	21	21	20	19	19	18	18	17	17	16	16	15	15	15	54
125	24	24	23	22	21	21	20	20	19	18	18	17	17	16	16	16	15	57
130	25	25	24	23	22	22	21	20	20	19	19	18	18	17	17	16	16	59
135	26	26	25	24	23	22	22	21	21	20	19	19	18	18	17	17	16	61
140	27	26	26	25	24	23	23	22	21	21	20	20	19	18	18	17	17	63
145	28	27	27	26	25	24	23	23	22	21	21	20	20	19	19	18	18	66
150	29	28	27	27	26	25	24	23	23	22	22	21	20	20	19	19	18	68
155	30	29	28	27	27	26	25	24	24	23	22	22	21	20	20	19	19	70
160	31	30	29	28	27	27	26	25	24	24	23	22	22	21	21	20	19	72
165	32	31	30	29	28	27	27	26	25	24	24	23	22	22	21	21	20	75
170	33	32	31	30	29	28	27	27	26	25	24	24	23	22	22	21	21	77
175	34	33	32	31	30	29	28	27	27	26	25	24	24	23	22	22	21	79
180	35	34	33	32	31	30	29	28	27	27	26	25	24	24	23	22	22	82
185	36	35	34	33	32	31	30	29	28	27	27	26	25	24	24	23	23	84
190	37	36	35	34	33	32	31	30	29	28	27	26	26	25	24	24	23	86
195	38	37	36	35	33	32	31	31	30	29	28	27	26	26	25	24	24	88
200	39	38	37	35	34	33	32	31	30	30	29	28	27	26	26	25	24	91
205	40	39	37	36	35	34	33	32	31	30	29	29	28	27	26	26	25	93
210	41	40	38	37	36	35	34	33	32	31	30	29	28	28	27	26	26	95
215	42	41	39	38	37	36	35	34	33	32	31	30	29	28	28	27	26	98
220	43	42	40	39	38	37	36	34	33	32	32	31	30	29	28	27	27	100
225	44	43	41	40	39	37	36	35	34	33	32	31	31	30	29	28	27	102
230	45	43	42	41	39	38	37	36	35	34	33	32	31	30	30	29	28	104
235	46	44	43	42	40	39	38	37	36	35	34	33	32	31	30	29	29	107
240	47	45	44	43	41	40	39	38	36	35	34	33	33	32	31	30	29	109
245	48	46	45	43	42	41	40	38	37	36	35	34	33	32	31	31	30	111
250	49	47	46	44	43	42	40	39	38	37	36	35	34	33	32	31	30	114

150 152.5 155 157.5 160 162.5 165 167.5 170 172.5 175 177.5 180 182.5 185 187.5 190

Height (centimetres)

□ **Underweight**   ▨ **Weight Appropriate**   ▨ **Overweight**   ■ **Obese**

---

23   Source:www.slim-fast.com. Adapted from The National Institute of Health. NHLBI Clinical Guidelines on Overweight and Obesity June 1998. www.nhlbi.nih.gov/guidelines.

Annex 3: Nutritional and energy requirements

Estimated Average Requirements[24]

Age	Males (kcal)	Females (kcal)	Age	Males (kcal)	Females (kcal)
0-3 mo	545	515	11-14 yr	2220	1845
4-6 mo	690	645	15-18 yr	2755	2110
7-9 mo	825	765	19-50 yr	2550	1940
10-12 mo	920	865	51-59 yr	2550	1900
1-3 yr	1230	1165	60-64 yr	2380	1900
4-6 yr	1715	1545	65-74 yr	2330	1900
7-10 yr	1970	1740	74+ yr	2100	1810

Fat, protein and carbohydrate are the three nutrients that provide energy. Alcohol also provides energy. There is some evidence to suggest that a poor energy mix of the diet is a risk factor in various diseases such as coronary heart disease and certain cancers. The COMA panel reviewed this evidence and concluded that it would be useful to set DRVs[25] for total fat (fatty acids and glycerol), fatty acids, sugars and starches (Table 3)

Suggested population averages for protein, carbohydrate and fat as a percentage of dietary energy

	Diet containing alcohol[26]	Diet not containing alcohol
Protein	15	15
Total Carbohydrate	47	50
Non milk extrinsic sugars[27]	10	11
Total fat	33	35
Saturated fatty acids	10	11
Polyunsaturated fatty acids	6[28]	6.5
Trans fatty acids	2	2
Monosaturated fatty acids	12	13

---

24 ww.nutrition.org.uk

25 DRVs – Dietary Reference Values; EAR – Estimated Average Requirements

26 Alcohol should provide no more than 5% of energy in the diet

27 NMES – free sugar not bound in foods, eg table sugar, honey and sugars in fruit juices, but excluding milk sugar.

28 An individual maximum of 10% applies (with an individual minimum of 0.2% from linolenic acid, and 1% linolenic acid).

Approximate daily intakes for adults aged 19–50

	Males	Females
Protein[29]	55.5g	45g
Total Carbohydrate[30]	320g	245g
Fat[31]	95g	70g
Saturates	30g	20g
Sodium	2.5g	2g
Fibre	20g	16g
Sugar	70g	50g

---

29 *Dietary Reference Values for Food Energy and Nutrients for the UK*, Department of Health, 1991

30 Figure for carbohydrate calculated for the Committee by the FSA. Carbohydrates have not been included in Guideline Daily Amounts because these were thought to be less important than other categories for which GDAs were given, and potentially misleading.

31 Guideline Daily Amounts for fat, saturates, sodium, fibre and sugar taken from Williams C, Rayner M, Myatt M, Boag A, *Use your label – making sense of nutrition information*, MAFF, 1996

Annex 4: Energy inputs and outputs

	Nutritional content:[33]		Minutes required to burn off by activity:[32]		
	Calories	Fat grams	walking slowly	walking mod. quickly	strenuous activity
Snack Food					
Mars Bar (65g)	294	11.4	98	59	39
Popcorn (100g)	405	7.7	135	81	54
Entrees					
Big Mac (215g)	492	23	164	98	66
Cheeseburger	379	18.9	126	76	51
Kentucky Fried Chicken (67g)	195	12	65	39	26
Hamburger (108g)	254	7.7	85	51	34
Pizza Deluxe (1 slice/66g)	171	6.7	57	34	23
Pizza (‰ pizza/135g)	263	4.9	88	53	35
Potato Wedges (135g)	279	13	93	56	37
Bombay Potato (200g)	202	10.4	67	40	27
Chicken Korma (300g)	498	31	166	100	66
Chicken Tikka (150g)	232	6.2	77	46	31
Beverages					
Can of coke (330ml)	139	0	46	28	19
Pint of beer	182	0	61	36	24
Gin, 40% alcohol (25ml)	55	0	18	11	7
Sherry (50ml)	68	0	23	14	9
Wine (1 glass/120ml)	87	0	29	17	12
Vodka, 40% alcohol (25ml)	55	0	18	11	7

32 Total energy used by a man aged 25 years (weighing 65kg) to do various activities. Source: Ministry of Agriculture, Fisheries and Food (1992) Manual of Nutrition. HMSO, London

33 Source: www.weightlossresources.co.uk.

Total energy used by a man aged 25 years (weighing 65kg) to undertake various activities.[34]

	Average energy expenditure[35] Kcal/min	Minutes to burn off a 65g Mars Bar (294cal) 294 cal/(Kcal/min)	Minutes to burn a 215g Big Mac (492cal) 494 cal/(Kcal/min)
Everyday Activities			
Sitting	1.40	210	351
Standing	1.70	173	289
Washing, dressing	3.50	84	141
Walking slowly	3.00	98	164
Walking moderately quickly	5.00	59	98
Walking up and down stairs	9.00	33	55
Work and Recreation			
Light Activity (most domestic work, golf, lorry driving, carpentry, bricklaying)	2.5-4.9	79	133
Moderate Activity (gardening, tennis, dancing, jogging, cycling up to 20km per hour, digging)	5.0-7.4	47	79
Strenuous Activity (coal mining, cross-country running, football, swimming [crawl])	>7.5	39	66

34 In 2002, the average man in England was 174.8 cm tall, weighed 82.4 kg and had a BMI of 26.9. The average woman was 161.3 cm tall, weighed 69.5 kg and had a BMI 26.7. See "Body mass index, by survey year, age and sex," Adults 1993-2002 Table 6, Health Survey for England – Trend Data.

35 Source: Ministry of Agriculture, Fisheries and Food (1992) Manual of Nutrition. HMSO, London.

List of Abbreviations

ACT	Activity Co-ordination Team
ASA	Advertising Standards Authority
BHF	British Heart Foundation
BMI	Body Mass Index
CAP	Common Agricultural Policy
CHD	Coronary Heart Disease
DCMS	Department for Culture, Media and Sport
DEFRA	Department for Environment, Food and Rural Affairs
DfES	Department for Education and Skills
DfT	Department for Transport
DoH	Department of Health
FSA	Food Standards Agency
HEA	Health Education Authority
HFCS	High Fructose Corn Syrup
IOTF	International Obesity Task Force
LTP	Local Transport Plan
NAO	National Audit Office
NICE	National Institute for Clinical Excellence
NSF	National Service Framework
ODPM	Office of the Deputy Prime Minister
OFCOM	Office of Communications
Ofsted	Office for Standards in Education
PCO	Primary Care Organisation
PCT	Primary Care Trust
PE	Physical Exercise
PSA	Public Service Agreement
RCGP	Royal College of General Physicians
RCP	Royal College of Physicians
SHA	Strategic Health Authority
TOAST	The Obesity Awareness and Solutions Trust
WHO	World Health Organization

Formal minutes

Thursday 10 May 2004

Members present:
Mr David Hinchliffe, in the Chair

Mr David Amess	Jim Dowd
John Austin	Mr Jon Owen Jones
Mr Keith Bradley	Dr Doug Naysmith
Mr Paul Burstow	Dr Richard Taylor

The Committee deliberated.

Draft Report (*Obesity*), proposed by the Chairman, brought up and read.

Ordered, That the Chairman's draft Report be read a second time, paragraph by paragraph.

Paragraphs 1 to 411 read and agreed to.

Summary agreed to.

An Annex (*The economic cost of obesity*) agreed to.

Another Annex (*Calculate your body mass index*) agreed to.

Another Annex (*Nutritional and energy requirements*) agreed to.

Another Annex (*Energy inputs and outputs*) agreed to.

Resolved, That the Report be the Third Report of the Committee to the House.

Ordered, That the Chairman do make the Report to the House.

Ordered, That the provisions of Standing Order No. 134 (Select Committees (Reports)) be applied to the Report.

[Adjourned till Thursday 6 May at 10.00 am.

Witnesses

Thursday 12 June 2003

Mr Mike Ash, Deputy Director, Planning Directorate, Office of the Deputy Prime Minister, **Ms Danila Armstrong**, Acting Nutrition Programme Manager, Cardiovascular Disease and Cancer Prevention, and **Ms Imogen Sharp**, Business Area Head, Department of Health, **Mrs Patricia Hayes**, Head, Charging and Local Transport Division, Department for Transport, **Mr Alec McGivan**, Director of Sport, Department for Culture, Media and Sport and **Ms Mela Watts**, Divisional Manager, Curriculum Division, Department for Education and Skills.   Ev 23

Thursday 26 June 2003

Professor Sir George Alberti, President, International Diabetes Federation, **Dr Geof Rayner**, Chairman, UK Public Health Association, **Professor Julian Peto**, Institute of Cancer Research, **Professor Hubert Lacey**, Royal College of Psychiatrists, **Professor Jane Wardle**, Health Behaviour Unit, University College, London and **Dr Tim Barrett**, Consultant Paediatric Endocrinologist, Birmingham Children's Hospital   Ev 58

Thursday 17 July 2003

Professor Andrew Prentice, MRC International Nutrition Group, London School of Hygiene and Tropical Medicine, **Dr Tim Lobstein**, Food Commission, **Professor Adrianne Hardmann**, Emeritus Professor, School of Sport and Exercise Sciences, University of Loughborough, **Dr Susan Jebb**, Head of Nutrition and Health Research, MRC Human Nutrition Research Centre and **Dr Nick Wareham**, Institute of Public Health, University of Cambridge.   Ev 85

Thursday 18 September 2003

Mr Len Almond, Director, British Heart Foundation, National Centre for Physical Activity and Health, Loughborough University, **Ms Jeanette Longfield**, Co-ordinator, Sustain, **Mr Paul Osborne**, Director, Safe Routes to Schools, Sustrans, **Ms Kath Dalmeny**, Research Officer, Food Commission and **Mr Paul Lincoln**, Chief Executive, National Heart Forum.   Ev 126

Thursday 30 October 2003

Professor Marion Nestle, Chair, Department of Nutrition, Food Studies and Public Health, New York University.   Ev 144

Thursday 6 November 2003

Dr Alan Maryon Davis, Faculty of Public Health, Royal College of Physicians, **Mr John Grimshaw**, Executive Director and Chief Engineer, Sustrans, **Professor Chris Riddoch**, Middlesex University, **Dr Sue Campbell**, Chief Executive, Youth Sport Trust and Chair, UK Sport and **Mr Tom Franklin**, Director, Living Streets   Ev 167

Thursday 13 November 2003

Mrs Cilla Snowball, Chief Executive, Abbott Mead Vickers—BBDO, **Mr Bruce Haines**, Group Chief Executive, Leo Burnett Ltd and **Mr Andrew Brown**, Director General, Advertising Association (also representing Food Advertising Unit).   Ev 199

Thursday 27 November 2003

Mr Andrew Cosslett, Director, Europe, Middle East and Africa Confectionery, Cadbury Schweppes, **Mr Julian Hilton-Johnson**, Vice-President, McDonald's Restaurants Ltd, **Mr Martin Glenn**, President, PepsiCo UK and **Mr Tim Mobsby**, Area President, Kellogg's Europe.   Ev 245

Thursday 4 December 2003

Mr Richard Ali, Director, Food Policy, British Retail Consortium, **Mr David Croft**, Head, Group Brand and Technology and **Mrs Susan Bromley**, Marketing Development Manager, The Co-operative Group, **Ms Penny Coates**, Director, Private Label, ASDA Stores Ltd and **Mr David North**, Director, Government Affairs, Tesco Plc.   Ev 280
Mr Barry Gardiner MP.   Ev 313

Thursday 18 December 2003

Dr Ian Campbell, Chairman, National Obesity Forum, **Dr Colin Waine**, Visiting Professor, Primary and Community Care, University of Sunderland, **Dr Nick Finer**, Hon. Consultant Physician, Obesity Medicine, Addenbrooke's Hospital NHS Trust, **Professor John Baxter**, Secretary, British Obesity Surgery Society and **Ms Dympna Pearson**, Chair, Dieticians in Obesity Management (UK).   Ev 337

Professor Iain Broom, Consultant in Clinical Biochemistry and Metabolic Medicine, Grampian University Hospitals Trust, **Ms Louise Mann**, Practice Nurse, **Ms Amanda Avery**, Community Dietician, Greater Derby Primary Care Trust, **Ms Sally Hayes**, Lead Nurse and **Ms Emma Croft**, Community Dietician, Leeds North West Primary Care Trust.   Ev 356

Ms Paula Hunt, Nutritionist and Dietician, Weight Watchers, **Dr Jacquie Lavin**, Nutritionist, Slimming World, **Ms Jackie Cox**, Joint Chair, The Obesity Awareness and Solutions Trust and **Dr Helen Truby**, Senior Lecturer, University of Surrey, Principal Investigator, BBC Diet Trials.   Ev 382

Thursday 8 January 2004

Ms Sue Davies, Principal Policy Adviser, Consumers' Association and **Dr Mike Rayner**, Director, British Heart Foundation Health Promotion Group.   Ev 394

Thursday 15 January 2004

Mr Callton Young, Head, Food and Drink Industry Division, Department for Environment, Food and Rural Affairs, **Mr Andrew Wadge**, Director, Food Safety Policy, **Mr Tom Murray**, Head, Nutrition Division, and **Ms Rosemary Hignett**, Head, Food Labelling and Standards Division, Food Standards Agency.   Ev 408

Thursday 11 March 2004

Miss Melanie Johnson MP, Parliamentary Under-Secretary of State for Public Health, **Ms Imogen Sharp**, Branch Head, Health Improvement and Prevention Team, **Ms Danila Armstrong**, Nutrition Programme Manager, and **Dr Adrienne Cullum**, Senior Nutrition Scientist, Department of Health.   Ev 424

Monday 29 March 2004

Rt Hon Margaret Hodge MP, Minister of State, Minister for Children, and **Ms Mela Watts,** Divisional Manager, Curriculum Division, Department for Education and Skills, **Rt Hon Tessa Jowell MP**, Secretary of State, and **Mr Paul Heron,** Head of Sports Division, Department for Culture, Media and Sport.   Ev 442

List of written evidence

List of appendices to the Report contained in Volume III

List of unprinted written evidence

Additional papers have been received from the following and have been reported to the House but to save printing costs they have not been printed and copies have been placed in the House of Commons library where they may be inspected by members. Other copies are in the Record Office, House of Lords and are available to the public for inspection. Requests for inspection should be addressed to the Record Office, House of Lords, London SW1. (Tel 020 7219 3074) hours of inspection are from 9:30am to 5:00pm on Mondays to Fridays.

Automatic Vending Association

Amateur Swimming Association

Department of Health

Infant and Dietetic Foods Association

Snack, Nut and Crisp Manufacturers' Association

Meat and Livestock Commission

Faculty of Public Health Medicine

Gillian Alderton

FMS Healthcare Ltd

Health Food Manufacturers' Association

The Sugar Bureau

Dr Peter Bundred and Professor Marion Hetherington

Obesity Management Association

Dr Krystyna Matyka

Federation of City Farms and Community Gardens

Periodical Publishers Association

Weightwatchers

Council of Heads of Medical Schools

The Biscuit Cake Chocolate & Confectionery Alliance

Professor David Benton

English Table Tennis Association

Rosemary Conley Diet and Fitness Clubs

British Gymnastics

National Heart Forum

Pixall Ltd

Anne Sheldon

Slim Fast Foods Limited

Living Streets

The Christchurch Obesity, Prevention Programme in Schools

The UK Weight Control Trial

Mr Andy Dixon

Canderel

Enuresis Resource and Information Centre

Slimming World

Mr Andrew Farmer

Dr C E Corney

Amanda Avery

Jackie Bushell

Cholesterol UK

Lloydspharmacy

Hilary Jackson

Reports from the Health Committee since 2001

The following reports have been produced by the Committee since the start of the 2001 Parliament. The reference number of the Government's response to the Report is printed in brackets after the HC printing number.

Session 2003–04

First Report	The Work of the Health Committee	HC 95
Second Report	Elder Abuse	HC 111

Session 2002–03

First Report	The Work of the Health Committee	HC 261
Second Report	Foundation Trusts	HC 395 (Cm 5876)
Third Report	Sexual Health	HC 69 (Cm 5959)
Fourth Report	Provision of Maternity Services	HC 464 (Cm 6140)
Fifth Report	The Control of Entry Regulations and Retail Pharmacy Services in the UK	HC 571 (Cm 5896)
Sixth Report	The Victoria Climbié Inquiry Report	HC 570 (Cm 5992)
Seventh Report	Patient and Public Involvement in the NHS	HC 697 (Cm 6005)
Eight Report	Inequalities in Access to Maternity Services	HC 696 (Cm 6140)
Ninth Report	Choice in Maternity Services	HC 796 (Cm 6140)

Session 2001–02

First Report	The Role of the Private Sector in the NHS	HC 308 (Cm 5567)
Second Report	National Institute for Clinical Excellence	HC 515 (Cm 5611)
Third Report	Delayed Discharges	HC 617 (Cm 5645)

Printed in the United Kingdom by The Stationery Office Limited
5/2004   970776   19585

ISBN 0-215-01737-4

9 780215 017376